MIND IN THE BALANCE

COLUMBIA SERIES IN SCIENCE AND RELIGION

THE COLUMBIA SERIES IN SCIENCE AND RELIGION

The Columbia Series in Science and Religion is sponsored by the Center for the Study of Science and Religion (CSSR) at Columbia University. It is a forum for the examination of issues that lie at the boundary of these two complementary ways of comprehending the world and our place in it. By examining the intersections between one or more of the sciences and one or more religions, the CSSR hopes to stimulate dialogue and encourage understanding.

ROBERT POLLACK
The Faith of Biology and the Biology of Faith

B. ALAN WALLACE, ED.
Buddhism and Science: Breaking New Ground

LISA SIDERIS
*Environmental Ethics, Ecological Theory, and Natural Selection:
Suffering and Responsibility*

WAYNE PROUDFOOT, ED.
*William James and a Science of Religions: Reexperiencing
The Varieties of Religious Experience*

MORTIMER OSTOW
*Spirit, Mind, and Brain: A Psychoanalytic Examination of
Spirituality and Religion*

B. ALAN WALLACE
Contemplative Science: Where Buddhism and Neuroscience Converge

PHILIP CLAYTON AND JIM SCHAAL, EDITORS
Practicing Science, Living Faith: Interviews with Twelve Scientists

B. ALAN WALLACE
Hidden Dimensions: The Unification of Physics and Consciousness

PIER LUIGI LUISI WITH THE ASSISTANCE OF ZARA HOUSHMAND
Mind and Life: Discussions with the Dalai Lama on the Nature of Reality

MIND
IN THE
BALANCE

MEDITATION IN SCIENCE,

BUDDHISM, & CHRISTIANITY

[ ]

B. Alan Wallace

COLUMBIA UNIVERSITY PRESS / NEW YORK

Columbia University Press
Publishers Since 1893
New York   Chichester, West Sussex
Copyright © 2009 Columbia University Press
All rights reserved

Library of Congress Cataloging-in-Publication Data
Wallace, B. Alan.
Mind in the balance : meditation in science, Buddhism, and Christianity / B. Alan
Wallace.
p.   cm. — (The Columbia series in science and religion)
Includes bibliographical references (p.   ) and index.
ISBN 978-0-231-14730-9 (cloth : alk. paper) — ISBN 978-0-231-51970-0 (electronic)
1. Meditation. 2. Meditation—Buddhism. 3. Meditation—Christianity. I. Title. II.
Series.
BL627.W33   2009
158.1′2—dc22   2008022867

Columbia University Press books are printed on permanent
and durable acid-free paper.

This book is printed on paper with recycled content.
Printed in the United States of America
c 10 9 8 7 6 5 4 3 2 1

References to Internet Web sites (URLs) were accurate at the time of writing. Neither
the author nor Columbia University Press is responsible for URLs that may have
expired or changed since the manuscript was prepared.

For Sarah and Troy, and all who are seeking
greater understanding and meaning in life

CONTENTS

PREFACE

In the fall of 2006, my stepdaughter, Sarah Volland, wrote to me with a request. She began by commenting that she was utterly content with her life as a whole, including her level of material prosperity. What she really wanted now was to improve the quality of her interior life and her mind, and she asked me to write a book that would offer guidance in this regard, and that she could eventually share with her son. She wanted a book that would benefit her family and anyone else seeking knowledge in order to bring their life to a whole new level.

She put this request to me not only because of our close relationship but also because of my unusual background in Eastern and Western approaches to understanding. Over the past thirty-eight years, I have been blessed with many profound personal teachers, including the Dalai Lama and other extraordinary contemplatives and masters of meditation. Ordained as a monk by the Dalai Lama, I trained for fourteen years in Buddhist monasteries in India, Tibet, Sri Lanka, and Switzerland. During my time as a monk and since, I have devoted years to solitary meditation in the Himalayan mountains, Buddhist monasteries, deserts, and in my home in California. In addition, I received my undergraduate education at Amherst College in physics and the philosophy of science, earned my doctorate in religious studies at Stanford University, then taught for four years in the Department of Religious Studies at the University of California, Santa Barbara. Since 1990, I have collaborated with multiple teams of research cognitive scientists at major universities, exploring the effects of meditation on mental and emotional balance and well-being, and have established the Santa Barbara Institute for Consciousness Studies to promote such research. Over the years, I have translated and written many books intended for Buddhist scholars and contemplatives, philosophers and scientists.

But Sarah asked me to write a book for readers like her, one that would address the fundamental questions about the nature of the mind and human existence without using the technical jargon of Buddhism, science, and philosophy. She wrote that when she was younger, she had always felt that she was born to do something truly great and meaningful, and she thought those feelings were unique to her. But through many friendships and relationships, she was surprised to discover that most of her close friends and companions had all had those same feelings, that they are here for a special purpose. But not many people seem to ever discover or fulfill that purpose. She felt there must be a reason that we have a calling for greatness, but unfortunately, those feelings fade with age and without good answers to our questions.

She has been a Christian for most of her life and feels that she has learned and experienced many great things from this religion. But she senses that there is much more to know and discover. And her deepest intuition tells her that meditation will be the purest and most profound form of prayer that she can experience. For this reason, she wishes to learn the truest and oldest forms of meditation, as well as the history and origins of those practices. By engaging in meditation, she hopes to find answers to questions we all ask: Who am I? Are we simply the roles we are currently playing in our lives, as parents, spouses, and members of society? Or is there much more to each of us on a deeper level, which is not just a product of our environment? Do we exist as anything other than our bodies? Are we born into sin and evil, and can human nature be transformed so that we are completely good and feel at one with God?

Knowing of my long collaboration in various research projects with cognitive scientists, she also asked what neuroscientists who have studied expert meditators have to say about their accomplishments. On the basis of such research, what accomplishments can we expect to reach in the modern world, given our current lifestyles? What levels might exist beyond that? And what benefits do ordinary people get when they meditate regularly? What problems do they encounter, and how do they overcome them? Can an agnostic benefit from meditation? Is there a quick-fix meditation version for busy people who are leery of any organized religion?

I was deeply moved by her request, and this book is what I have to offer in response, drawing from the wisdom of my many teachers and mentors in the East and the West, including Buddhist and Christian scholars and contemplatives, philosophers, psychologists, neuroscientists, and physicists. I have found greater joy in writing this book than in anything else I've written. I would write a chapter and send it to Sarah for her review. She would read with a critical eye, often asking for clarification of difficult points, additional material that I had not thought of, revision of sections she felt were not well expressed, and deletion of material she thought was irrelevant. In all the writing I've done over the past thirty-five years, I've never had a better editor, one who was so deeply interested in the material, so supportive of my efforts to share what I had learned, yet who never flinched from offering pointed criticism whenever she felt my writing was unsatisfactory.

Following the opening chapters on the origins of meditation and scientific studies of its benefits, part II presents a sequence of paired chapters focusing on meditative practices and their related theories. The chapters on practice are intended to provide an overview of a gradual path of meditations that are equally relevant to and compatible with both Christianity and Buddhism. They begin with the most rudimentary training in mindfulness and culminate in the most advanced practices designed to fathom the innermost nature of consciousness and its relation to the world at large. Readers wishing to explore these practices may do so by reading the instructions and then trying them out, or they may purchase a CD of recorded instructions for each technique to listen to while learning how to practice. This CD is available from the Santa Barbara Institute for Consciousness Studies (http://sbinstitute.com). Those who venture into this sequence of meditations should not expect to experience the results of all of them simply by trying them a few times. The full benefits can normally be gained only with years of rigorous practice under the guidance of a qualified teacher.

I am deeply grateful to Sarah for her initial request and for her unflagging efforts to help me respond to the best of my ability. I am also indebted to Kimberley Snow for her editorial suggestions, to both Kimberley Snow and Nancy Lynn Kleban for their excellent proofreading, and to Fred Cooper, Adam Frank, Ben Shapiro, and Pier Luigi Luisi for their advice on technical points. I especially wish to thank my friend and colleague Brian Hodel for his selfless efforts in polishing the manuscript as a whole. Finally, my sincere thanks go to Wendy Lochner, the religion and philosophy editor at Columbia University Press, who has been so supportive of my work, and to Leslie Kriesel, Assistant Managing Editor, for her excellent work of editing the entire manuscript. I hope that our efforts together will indeed be of benefit to those many people who are seekers of understanding and who wish to find greater meaning and fulfillment in their lives.

MIND IN THE BALANCE

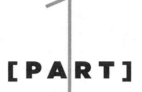

[PART]

MEDITATION: WHERE IT STARTED
AND HOW IT GOT HERE

Meditation is one of humanity's best-kept secrets. If beings from another galaxy were to study us closely—reading our history books, watching our movies, scouring the Internet—they would get only the most superficial understanding of it. They would conclude the same thing most of us believe about meditation: it is a relaxation technique good for relieving stress and as a secondary therapy for certain illnesses. And—oh yes—certain religions (Hinduism, Buddhism, and a few others) use it as part of worship. And that's all there is to it!

What's been hidden is meditation's role as a precision tool for exploring consciousness and the universe scientifically—that is, using empirical methods similar to those intrinsic to the scientific method. Since ancient times, meditators in different contemplative communities across the globe have systematically explored and reported their findings on inner reality and its connections to outer phenomena. Yes, they also discovered that meditation helped one attain a calm, serene lifestyle and had positive effects on mental and physical health. But these were only secondary benefits of their primary quest.

If some of these contemplatives deliberately kept their discoveries secret, the main reason the true origins of meditation remain hidden from the public today stems from the crude way we define "religion." We generally think of religion as simply an attitude based on faith in authority ("Jesus or Mohammed or Moses said 'X,' so I believe 'X.'"), and carelessly lump together those who believe without question the revelations of religious authorities and "religious groups" that question and explore in hopes of confirming and directly experiencing spiritual phenomena. There is a huge difference between the two. When we carefully examine them, we realize that regarding these two types of "religious" practitioners as identical makes as much sense as saying that the sun and the moon are the same because they are both in space.

This book presents a multicultural view of meditation—as a means for improving one's lifestyle; a way to achieve deep insights into the nature of the mind and consciousness, resulting in unprecedented well-being; and as a basis for genuine altruism and compassion. Part I outlines the history and development of meditation, demonstrating its principal goals and methods and how it differs from purely faith-based religion. If this difference is not understood and taken into account, it will be difficult to discern the importance and enormous potential of contemplation for healing our troubled and divided world.

1

WHO AM I?

In the ancient story of the blind men and the elephant,[1] a king gathered a group of men who were born blind and told them to examine an elephant and then describe what they found. One of them felt its head, while others individually touched its tusks, trunk, feet, and back. Depending on the part of the elephant they had touched, one by one, these blind men described it as being like a pot, a ploughshare, a rope, a pillar, and a wall. When they heard each other's different accounts, they immediately began debating and quarreling about who was right, some of them resorting to violence.

I am reminded of this story when I reflect on the variety of often conflicting answers given for the age-old question, who am I? Theologians, philosophers, and scientists have been trying to answer it for centuries, but only rarely have they agreed. How come? Could it be that their own particular biases have clouded the picture? Have their conditioned responses, their preferred sources of authority and methods of inquiry created a barrier to understanding?

We humans have had plenty of time to reflect upon our own identity. The Bible says that man is created in the image of God. If that's true, this must be a good thing, for the Bible insists that God is good and that his creation is good. But there are plenty of Jews and Christians who emphasize man's evil nature and our need to look outside of ourselves—to God or Jesus—for salvation from our innate defilements. There is abundant evidence throughout history and in today's world to support the assertion that humans are essentially evil. But there's no denying that there's a lot of good in the world too. So which is more basic, evil or good? Or are we simply a mixture of both? Theologians have been debating these points for centuries, with no resolution in sight.

Biologists tell us that humans have slowly evolved by a process of natural selection from earlier primates. From one generation to the next, the species that are alive now have gradually adapted to their changing environments so that they could continue to survive and procreate. If an individual survives long enough to bear offspring, it's an evolutionary success. If not, regardless of what it's done during the course of its life, it's a biological failure. So from a biologist's perspective, humans are animals, leading our lives under the influence of our genes, instincts, and emotions, with the prime directive of *survive and procreate*. The words "good" and "evil" don't mean anything scientifically, except insofar as they pertain to our ability to stay alive and make babies.

When psychiatrists, starting with Sigmund Freud, have addressed the issue of human nature, they have also emphasized our primitive drives for sex and domination over others. Their views tie in closely with those of evolutionary biologists and psychologists: while our conscious behavior may appear quite civilized and at times even altruistic, our subconscious impulses are dark, selfish, and brutal. But cognitive scientists are not completely in agreement on this point. Over the past ten years, the branch called "positive psychology" has arisen, which focuses on human flourishing and virtue. It's a young field of scientific inquiry, not yet backed by much hard empirical evidence. But these psychologists are raising important questions and expanding the horizons of their field, which has focused for the past sixty years almost entirely on the mentally ill, brain-damaged, and people with normal mental health. Only recently have they begun to explore the highest potentials of the human mind.

For much of the first half of the twentieth century, academic psychology in the United States was dominated by behaviorism, which insisted on studying human nature only through the examination of animal and human behavior. Behavioral scientists made a point of avoiding introspection—the firsthand exploration of our own minds and personal experience. Then in the 1960s, as behaviorism began to decline, cognitive psychology appeared, seeming to take subjective experience more seriously. But this was also the time when computer technology was on the rise, so researchers in this field were quick to compare the mind to a computer.

During the closing decades of the twentieth century, advances in technology allowed the brain sciences to progress like never before, and since then, many neuroscientists have come to the conclusion that the mind is really the brain, or the mind is what the brain does. They claim that all our personal experience consists of brain functions, influenced by the rest of the body, DNA, diet, behavior, and the environment. In the final analysis, human beings are biologically programmed robots, implying that we have essentially no more freedom of will than any other automata. Our programs are simply more complex than those of man-made machines. But not all neuroscientists agree. Some are now exploring the effects of thoughts and behavior on the brain. Even they generally regard the mind as an emergent property of the brain, so what they are saying is that some functions of the brain influence other functions. To date, however, there is no clear consensus about the implications of the research conducted so far.

You may have noticed that in all those approaches, something crucial has been left out: our own personal experience of what it's like to be a human being. Contemplatives in the East and the West, however, have explored the nature of the mind, consciousness, and human identity, and I believe they have illuminated dimensions of reality that remain largely unexplored in the modern world. Religion has become so hung up on doctrine, and science so materialistic, that contemplative methods of inquiry are often overlooked. And in the modern world, even when meditation is practiced, it's often used simply to alleviate stress and to overcome other physical and psychological problems. But meditation may also yield some of the deepest insights we can possibly gain about human nature and identity.

In terms of our individual sense of who we are, most of us identify strongly with the roles we play in everyday life, for example, parent, spouse, child, student, or person in a certain profession. Such roles are important, and they define us in our interrelations in society. But apart from our specific relations to other people and the kinds of activities we engage in on a regular basis, what's left over? Who are we when we sit quietly in our rooms, doing nothing but being present?

Let's approach this question practically by setting out on a kind of expedition into the frontiers of the mind. I especially like the word "expedition" because of its roots. It derives from the Latin word *expeditio,* made up of the syllable *ex,* which has the connotation of "coming out" or "freeing oneself," and *ped,* which means "feet." So "expedition" has the connotation of extricating ourselves from a place in which our feet are stuck. The kind of expedition I have in mind is one in which we first recognize where we are stuck in old ruts leading nowhere, and then take steps to free ourselves.

We are living in a frenzied world in which most of us think if we're not *doing something,* even watching TV, we're wasting time. We get so caught up in our activities, relationships, thoughts, and emotions that we think that's all there is to us. Let's take a brief time out. Find a quiet place in your home and a comfortable chair to sit in for ten minutes. Without deliberately thinking about anything, see if you can simply be aware of your body and mind. Be silent, and, without reacting, let the sensations of your body and thoughts and emotions arise to your awareness.

Tick, tick, tick, tick. . . .

Can you truly be mentally silent when you want to, or does your mind obsessively spew out one thought after another? When thoughts arise, can you simply observe them, or do you find yourself compulsively caught up in them, your attention captivated by each mental image and desire? Is this mind of yours really under your control, or is it controlling you, causing you to confuse your thoughts about the world with your immediate experience of your body, mind, and environment? A calm and clear mind can be put to great use, but one that is turbulent and out of control can do great harm to ourselves and others. So the first task on the path of contemplation is to harness the enormous power of the mind and turn it to good service.

THE ORIGINS OF CONTEMPLATION

CONTEMPLATION IN THE WEST

Throughout this book I shall refer to theories and practices of contemplation stemming primarily from ancient Greek philosophy, Christianity, and Buddhism. As we shall see, although each of these traditions has unique qualities, they have important similarities. The English word "contemplation" derives from the Latin *contemplatio,* which corresponds to the Greek *theoria.* Both terms refer to a total devotion to revealing, clarifying, and making manifest the nature of reality. Nowadays, "contemplation" usually means thinking about something. But the original meanings of "contemplation" and "theory" had to do with a direct perception of reality, not by the five physical senses or by thinking, but by mental perception.[1] For example, when you directly observe your own thoughts, mental images, and dreams, you are using mental perception, which can be refined and extended through the practice of contemplation. How then does meditation relate to contemplation? The Sanskrit word *bhavana* corresponds to the English word "meditation," and it literally means "cultivation." To meditate means to cultivate an understanding of reality, a sense of genuine well-being, and virtue. So *meditation* is a gradual process of training the mind, and it leads to the goal of *contemplation*, in which one gains insight into the nature of reality.

Within the Greek tradition, the practice of meditation can be traced back at least as far as Pythagoras (c. 582–507 B.C.E.), who was influenced by the Orphic religion and mysteries, which were focused on freeing the mind from impurities and opening up its deeper resources. Pythagoras was the first to call himself a *philosopher*, "one who loves wisdom," humbly rejecting the term *sophos*, or "wise man." And in his wide travels throughout the Mediterranean region and beyond, he did indeed seek wisdom, understanding.

In about 525 B.C.E., after a search of many years, Pythagoras moved from the Greek island of Samos to the city of Crotone in southern Italy. There he established a religious philosophical society in which he trained men and women to lead a life well balanced in body and spirit while living in a community of self-reliant communism. In order to purify their souls, they were required to maintain high ethical standards, engage in physical exercise, practice celibacy, follow a vegetarian diet, and engage in protracted periods of silence and various kinds of abstinence. Their formal education consisted of training in music, mathematics, astronomy, and meditation. Because none of Pythagoras's texts survives, we know little about the various kinds of meditation he and his followers taught and practiced.

Pythagoras is perhaps most renowned for the Pythagorean theorem, which pertains to the relative lengths of the three sides of a right triangle. Since this theorem had already been formulated in the eighth century B.C.E. in India,[2] it is possible that in his many travels, Pythagoras may have learned this and other branches of knowledge, especially pertaining to meditation, from Indian sources. He is also well known for his belief in reincarnation, according to which the soul is immortal and is reborn in both human and animal bodies. Legend has it that he claimed to be able to recall up to twenty of his own and others' past lives. But we have no way of knowing whether his alleged memories were accurate, and if they were, whether he was born with this ability or achieved it through meditation. One of the quotes attributed to Pythagoras is "Learn to be silent. . . . Let your quiet mind listen and absorb," and a primary focus of this meditative tradition was attending to the "harmony of the spheres," which combined themes from music, mathematics, and astronomy. He believed that the highest life is one devoted to *passionate, sympathetic contemplation,* which produced a kind of ecstasy coming from direct insight into the nature of reality.

The possible Indian origins of the Pythagorean theorem and his belief in reincarnation have led some historians to conclude that Pythagoras may have been influenced by ideas from India, transmitted via Persia and Egypt. We owe most of what we know about the Pythagoreans to Aristotle (384–322 B.C.E.). According to him, the Pythagoreans were the first to advance the study of mathematics, and to them all things in nature were modeled after numbers. Indeed, numbers were the first things in the whole of nature and pervaded everything. They conceived of numbers in terms of different configurations of units in space, and concluded on this basis that the elements of numbers are the elements of all things. According to Aristotle, "the Pythagoreans also believe in one kind of number—the mathematical; only they say it is not separate but sensible substances are formed out of it. For they construct the whole universe out of numbers—only not numbers consisting of abstract units; they suppose the units to have spatial magnitude."[3]

Pythagoras was said to have admired Judaism, in which God is seen as the one supreme ruler of the universe, on which he imposes his divine laws. According to the Jewish historian Flavius Josephus (37–c. 100 C.E.), the Jewish sect called the Essenes likewise admired the teachings of Pythagoras, for they followed a way of life modeled after his society.[4] Members of this sect lived in Judea from the mid-second century B.C.E. until 70 C.E., when they were destroyed by the Romans. Like the early Pythagoreans, the Essenes retreated from mainstream society, lived very frugally, shared communal property, and believed that God was best worshipped not by means of animal sacrifices but by purifying their minds. Although celibacy was not part of the Hebrew tradition, the Essenes shunned marriage—it posed a threat to communal life—but did not condemn it in principle. They engaged in ritual baths in cold water, or baptism, and believed in a healing ministry in which power came through the hands. Deeply critical of the ethical norms of the Jewish and Roman societies of their time, they believed that the kingdom of God was soon to come and would be heralded by a cataclysmic war between the righteous and the sinful.

Since the nineteenth century, scholars have speculated on the possible connection between the Essenes and John the Baptist as well as Jesus, which would imply that Pythagorean practices and beliefs influenced the early Christian tradition. Indeed, John the Baptist's lifestyle and teachings were remarkably similar to those of the Essenes. Leading a celibate life, wearing clothes made of camel's hair, and living on an ascetic diet of locusts and wild honey, he preached in the Desert of Judea, "Repent, for the kingdom of heaven is near." Like the Essenes, he baptized others as a ritual cleansing of their impurities and sins. When approached by Pharisees and Sadducees, he was harshly critical, calling them a brood of vipers.[5]

Foremost of all the Jews who came to John for baptism was Jesus of Nazareth, who praised him above all the prophets before him, saying, "Among those born of women there has not risen anyone greater than John the Baptist; yet he who is least in the kingdom of heaven is greater than he."[6] Since Jesus was baptized by John, we may assume he accepted John's teachings, and immediately following his baptism, Jesus left for the wilderness, where he fasted and prayed for forty days, during which he overcame the temptations of the devil. When he emerged from his desert solitude, he began to preach a message common to the Essenes and John the Baptist: "Repent, for the kingdom of heaven is near."[7]

Even if Flavius Josephus was correct in asserting that the Essenes followed a way of life taught to the Greeks by Pythagoras, it is difficult to know the extent to which the Essenes adopted Pythagorean beliefs such as reincarnation, though they also clearly believed in the immortality of the soul. It is remarkable, though, that Jesus declared John the Baptist to be the prophet Elijah.[8] This did not apparently startle his listeners, for many Jews already believed that the prophets might be reincarnated, or "resurrected." According to the Bible, while still alive, Elijah was taken up by a chariot of fire and horses of fire and brought to heaven in a whirlwind.[9] The New Testament declared that John was imbued with Elijah's "spirit and power," which could easily be interpreted as his being a reincarnation of Elijah. But theologians have interpreted these passages in various ways.

Teachings of the Pythagoreans, by way of Socrates (c. 470–399 B.C.E.) and Plato (c. 427–347 B.C.E.), were eventually assimilated into the philosophical school of Neoplatonism, which was founded by Plotinus (c. 205–270). Born in Egypt, he immersed himself in Greek thought for nine years in Alexandria, and then joined an expedition to Persia in the hopes of studying the philosophical writings of the Persians and Indians. But this military venture failed, and he never reached his destination. Plotinus believed human perfection and happiness were attainable in this world and could be achieved through the practice of contemplation. The goal was to achieve ecstatic union with the One, which he taught was the ultimate reality, transcending all words and concepts. His famous work *Enneads* was compiled, arranged, and edited by Porphyry (c. 232–305) (also known for his *Life of Pythagoras*), who related that Plotinus attained such divine union four times during the six years Porphyry studied with him. Contemplation is the single "thread" that unites the One with all created things, which emerge from it, and by the practice of contemplation one comes to know the source of one's own being. Like Pythagoras and Socrates, Plotinus believed that individual souls reincarnate, experiencing the results of their ethical and unethical behavior from lifetime to lifetime until finally they are utterly purified and find the highest happiness born of contemplation.

Over the centuries, Plotinus's writings have inspired Christian, Jewish, Muslim, and Gnostic philosophers and contemplatives, one of the most influential of whom was Origen (c. 185–254). Born in Alexandria, he was widely viewed as the greatest Christian theologian of his time. He, too, believed the soul evolves spiritually from lifetime to lifetime, until it finally advances to knowledge (*gnosis*) of God by means of contemplation (*theoria*). Beginning in about the third century, Christian contemplatives began to take up the solitary, meditative life in the Sahara desert of Egypt. Many took refuge there after they fled from the chaos and persecution of the Roman Empire. These original desert hermits, known as Desert Fathers, formed communities at the edges of population centers, far enough away to be safe from imperial scrutiny, but still close enough to have access to civilization.[10]

Although most of the early Desert Fathers were illiterate, Evagrius of Pontus (345–399) was a highly educated classical scholar, and he was one of the first of the Desert Fathers to begin recording and systematizing their oral teachings. Evagrius was a staunch supporter of Origen and embraced his views about the reincarnation of human souls and their final perfection in union with God. One of his principal disciples, John Cassian (c. 360–433), adapted Evagrius's works for his Western students and established the Abbey of St. Victor, a complex of two monasteries, one for men and the other for women, in southern France. This was one of the first such institutes in the West, and it served as a model for the later development of Christian monasticism.

CONTEMPLATION IN THE EAST

The earliest evidence for a meditative culture anywhere in the world is found in the Indus valley civilization that stretched from what is now Pakistan to the Ganges valley in India, and reached its peak during the period 3000 to 2500 B.C.E. Thousands of carved seals in the form of small clay tablets have been preserved from this civilization, containing some of the world's oldest writings. A few of those seals depict yogis sitting in classic meditative postures.

There are surprisingly few literary references to meditation before the time of Gautama the Buddha (c. 563–483 B.C.E.), who was a contemporary of Pythagoras. But it is clear that there was already a very rich and diverse tradition of contemplation in which he immersed himself as soon as he left his palatial home at the age of twenty-nine. He devoted himself to a life of contemplative inquiry in order to escape from the cycle of birth, death, and rebirth, so belief in reincarnation appears to have been common in his day. His first meditation teacher was Alara Kalama, who was proficient in *samadhi,* or meditative states in which the attention is withdrawn from the physical senses, thoughts are calmed, and one experiences extraordinary bliss and serenity. Since, according to Buddhist accounts, the type of meditation he taught can lead to direct, reliable knowledge of past lives, advanced meditators regarded reincarnation not as a matter of religious belief but as an empirically verifiable truth.

According to early Buddhist records, Gautama swiftly achieved the most sublime, rarified samadhi taught by Alara Kalama, in which his mind entered a formless dimension of existence devoid of all content except an experience of pure nothingness. But this did not satisfy his aspirations for liberation from the cycle of existence, so he sought out an even more accomplished contemplative named Uddaka Ramaputta, under whose guidance he achieved an even subtler samadhi. But Gautama recognized that such states of meditative absorption alone did not yield his goal of "the supreme state of sublime peace" through knowing reality as it is. For he found that after one emerges from such meditation and engages with the everyday world, one is still prone to suffering and its underlying causes. When he recognized that achieving these states didn't get to the root of the problem, Gautama spent years tormenting his body with ascetic practices, including fasting. His aim was to attain liberation by achieving a kind of mastery of mind over matter. But the end result was that his body became emaciated and his mental faculties were impaired. He then realized that achieving samadhi was not an ultimate goal, but such refined states of consciousness could be used for meditatively investigating the nature of suffering and its causes.

Among the great religious teachers throughout history, the Buddha is unique in discouraging belief that something is true simply because many people say it's true, or because it's based on long-standing tradition, scriptural authority, hearsay, speculation, or reverence for a teacher. Rather, to the best of one's ability, one should put others' claims to the test of one's own experience and judge for oneself. It stands to reason, then, that this is precisely what the Buddha did regarding claims of reincarnation that were prevalent during his time.[11] In the earliest records of his narration of his achievement of enlightenment, he describes how, with his mind concentrated, purified, malleable, and calm, he achieved "direct knowledge" of the nature of consciousness and the roots of suffering.[12] His first direct knowledge was of the specific circumstances of many thousands of his own former lives over the course of many eons of world contraction and expansion. His second direct knowledge was the contemplative observation of the succession of lifetimes of other beings, ascertaining the relations between their deeds and their effects as they played out in subsequent lives. And his third direct knowledge on the night of his enlightenment was his realization of the Four Noble Truths: "I had direct knowledge, as it actually is, that 'This is suffering,' that 'This is the origin of suffering,' that 'This is the cessation of suffering,' and that 'This is the way leading to the cessation of suffering.'" It was at this point that Gautama became a buddha, an "awakened one," due to his mind being utterly freed from all afflictions and obscurations. In this realization of nirvana he found the supreme state of sublime peace that he had been seeking, and he devoted the remaining forty-five years of his life to leading other people to such freedom from suffering. For this reason he came to be known as the "Great Physician," who showed how to realize genuine well-being through purifying the mind of its afflictions, cultivating virtue, and gaining contemplative insight into the nature of reality.

In this very brief survey of the origins of meditation in Greek philosophy, Christianity, and Buddhism, there are a number of common themes and insights. But the orientation of meditative practice is different for each tradition, as are the interpretations of contemplative experience. The Pythagoreans believed in an orderly universe, and though they probably accepted classical Greek polytheism, they believed in one superior divinity above all others. For them, meditation was closely related to music, mathematics, and astronomy. For the Christians, it was focused on union with the one supreme God, and for the Buddhists, who shared the Indian belief in the existence of many gods, meditation was for the purpose of achieving liberation from the cycle of existence. But in the beginning and later development of each of these traditions, it is apparent that meditation played a vital role.

THE SCIENTIFIC EXTERNALIZATION
OF MEDITATION

Although contemplation lies at the root of Western religions, philosophy, and science, it plays hardly any role in science today. This is not the result of a gradual decline, as in Christianity, but rather can be traced back to the origins of modern science in the seventeenth century. At that time, the supernatural world—consisting of God and other spiritual entities such as the devil and angels, heaven and hell—was to be accepted on the basis of the authority of the Bible. Theologians were in charge of understanding this domain of reality, and their views were accepted on faith. The human soul could be regarded as spiritual in the sense that it came from God and has free will, independent of the body and physical environment. But it is also natural in the sense that it governs the body and is influenced by the physical senses. So the spiritual aspects of the soul were to be accepted on *faith,* as coming from divine authority, and its natural aspects were explained by philosophers who relied principally on their powers of *reasoning.* Scientists had the task of understanding the third domain of reality—the external world of matter and natural forces—on the basis of direct observations and experiments.

The word "meditation" can be traced back to the Indo-European verbal root "med," which means to "consider" or "measure." As we've seen, in early Christianity, meditation was an experiential means for gaining direct, contemplative insight into the nature of reality. But in medieval scholasticism and modern philosophy, meditation was reduced to rational, introspective considerations. Aiming to understand the external universe of matter, science has devised its own "meditations" in the form of measurements of physical processes that can be validated by all competent observers.

All the great pioneers of science in the seventeenth century were devout Christians, and their inquiries into the world of nature could be seen as a mystical attempt to merge man's understanding of the natural world with the understanding of God. Christian contemplatives from the time of Augustine had sought this same goal, and they had assumed that it could not be realized in this life, only in heaven. As inward-looking contemplative inquiry in Europe diminished, scientists devised new methods of outward-looking inquiry, which they hoped would lead to divine understanding in this life.

Among these innovators, none was more influential than Galileo Galilei (1564–1642). As a child, Galileo entered a monastery of the Camaldolese order, which combined the solitary life of the hermit with the strict life of the monk. He was attracted to this lifestyle and wanted to join the order, but his father wouldn't let him, for he couldn't afford to support his son in a religious vocation that generated no income. Obeying his father's wish, Galileo entered the University of Pisa to study medicine, but soon shifted to mathematics and science. On the whole, he despised scholastic philosophy, which he saw as nothing more than an entrenched conservatism that was suspicious of innovative ideas and novel methods of inquiry.

Galileo was largely responsible for laying the foundations of the "scientific method" for studying the material world: sophisticated, rigorous, quantitative observations of physical entities, combined with mathematical analysis of the observed data. The motivation behind his research was to understand the nature of God's creation from God's own perspective, transcending the limitations and illusions of the human senses. This could be done, he proposed, by using mathematical reasoning, for he believed that mathematics was God's own language. This theistic interpretation of the central role of mathematics in nature had been advocated centuries earlier by the Pythagoreans.

While Galileo was content to leave supernatural questions in the hands of the Church, he insisted that the scientific study of the natural world must proceed freely and independently of the authority of the Bible and Greek thought. In taking this revolutionary step, he reversed the medieval scholastic hierarchy of knowledge. Empirical observation, which philosophers generally held to be the lowest form of knowledge, was raised to the highest level. Reason was important for interpreting empirical findings, and the authority of tradition was accepted only as long as it was not contradicted by rigorous observation or sound reasoning. What an enormous shift!

Galileo abandoned the Aristotelian emphasis on understanding *why* things are the way they are and focused instead on painstaking observations and measurements of *how* celestial and terrestrial objects move. The scholastic philosophers of his time uncritically accepted Aristotle's views that celestial bodies were unchanging and moved in perfect circles, with the Earth at their center. In 1609, Galileo created a telescope with the power to magnify images twenty times, and with this new instrument he discovered four moons of Jupiter (which revolved around Jupiter, not the Earth), craters on the Moon, sunspots (showing that celestial bodies were not immutable), and the phases of Venus, which indicated that it revolved around the Sun, not the Earth. Other astronomers with inferior instruments complained of not being able to confirm all his observations. As a result, some of them questioned their validity, while others went so far as to claim that they were optical illusions created by Galileo's lenses.

Medieval astronomers had long been familiar with the deceptive nature of the appearances of celestial bodies, especially when it came to the apparent motion of the planets. In accordance with ancient Greek thought, they assumed that the Moon, Sun, planets, and stars all revolved in perfect circles around the Earth. During a single night, planets are seen to move across the sky from east to west, but if observed from one night to the next, they usually appear to move from west to east against the background stars. Occasionally, however, a planet's motion will appear to reverse direction, and for a short time it will move from east to west against the background constellations. This reversal is known as "retrograde motion." To explain such deceptive appearances so that they accorded with Greek thought, early astronomers devised a complicated, abstract system of epicycles, whereby the planets moved around small circular paths that in turn made larger circular orbits around the Earth. This, they believed, was the real, objective motion of the planets in contrast to the false, subjective appearances of their retrograde motion. This entire theory turned out to be based on false assumptions, and it was only with the use of the telescope, focused on the deceptive appearances of celestial bodies, that the science of astronomy could progress.

When Galileo first presented his discoveries through his telescope as supporting evidence for the Copernican theory that the Earth revolved around the Sun, it was not the Church that attacked him. In fact, Jesuit and Dominican priests and bishops delighted in the new vistas the telescope opened up, and they threw luxuriant parties for Galileo in Rome to celebrate his new discoveries. Father Clavius, who was the undisputed leader of Jesuit astronomy, at first had a hard time accepting these findings. But once he and his colleagues had obtained telescopes of their own, they corroborated all of Galileo's observations. What eventually drew the Church into conflict with Galileo were its lay academic advisors, who insisted that Rome had a duty to stop Galileo, for if he were left unchecked, he would destroy the entire university system by undermining the Aristotelian beliefs on which it was based. These scholastic philosophers refused to even look through a telescope, for they adamantly insisted that whatever was seen through the lenses that contradicted their beliefs had to be optical illusions.

Galileo's discoveries using his telescope transformed the controversy about the relative movements of the Sun and Earth from an intellectual debate to a question that might be decided on the basis of evidence. He prided himself on having been the first to build a proper telescope and point it toward the sky, but he most valued his genius in making careful observations of a wide range of physical entities, understanding the behavior of their parts, and describing these in terms of mathematical proportions.[1]

While Galileo is regarded as the father of modern science for his role in establishing the scientific method of inquiry, the French philosopher, mathematician, and scientist René Descartes (1596–1650) has been dubbed the father of modern philosophy for presenting the conceptual framework in which scientific inquiry would be conducted. After earning a law degree in accordance with his father's wish, Descartes abandoned academic life and resolved to seek no knowledge other than that which could be found in himself or else in the "great book of the world."[2] While traveling in Germany at the age of twenty, thinking about using mathematics to solve problems in physics, he had a vision in a dream through which he "discovered the foundations of a marvelous science." This became a pivotal point in young Descartes' experience, and he dedicated the rest of his life to investigating the connection between mathematics and nature.

The foundation of Descartes' science was the proposition that objects have two kinds of qualities. As *spatially extended substances,* all physical objects have length, height, breadth, change, location, duration, and number, and by way of these *primary qualities,* they can be understood in terms of mathematics. Objects also have what are called *secondary qualities,* such as color, sound, taste, smell, heat, and cold. He believed that these qualities do not exist objectively in physical objects themselves, but are rather qualities of our perception of the world around us. When "clearly and distinctly perceived," he concluded that objective, primary qualities could be known decisively. In contrast, when it came to secondary qualities, he commented, "they are to be found in my thought with such obscurity and confusion that I do not know even whether they are true, or false and only apparent, that is to say, whether the ideas I form of these qualities are truly the ideas of real things, or whether they represent to me only [ideas] which cannot exist."[3]

Descartes suggested that the distinction between primary and secondary qualities of matter is necessary in order to avoid drawing false conclusions about the nature of reality. Specifically, he was refuting the assumption commonly known as "naïve realism" that we all carry from childhood—that colors, sounds, smells, tastes, and tactile sensations exist in the objective world, independently of our perceptions.[4] He concluded, "It can be shown that weight, color, and all other such qualities which are sensed in bodily matter, can be taken away from it, while leaving the matter itself intact. From which it follows that its nature depends on none of these."[5] The objective world, in Descartes' view, is actually colorless, odorless, tasteless, and so on. The refutation of naïve realism accords with all subsequent scientific discoveries and remains integral to the scientific view of nature as a whole. While elementary particles, atoms, molecules, electromagnetic fields, and waves are believed to exist independently of any observer, the *visual images* we perceive of the world around us do not exist out there. As neurologist Antonio Damasio comments, "There is no picture of the object being transferred from the object to the retina and from the retina to the brain."[6] Such pictures exist only in our minds, wherever they are.

The word "science" stems from the Indo-European verbal root *sker,* which means to "cut" or "separate," and under Descartes' direction, modern science began by drawing a sharp boundary separating the objective world of the physical universe from the subjective worlds of individuals' personal experience. In making this absolute separation between the objective physical world and the subjective world of the mind, Descartes, in effect, turned the material world over to scientists and left the subjective world to philosophers and theologians. Ever since the time of Galileo and Descartes, generations of physicists and biologists have followed this distinction and have made extraordinary progress in measuring and understanding objective, physical, quantifiable realities. In fact, by the closing decades of the nineteenth century, many physicists believed their understanding of the physical world was complete and perfect in all main respects. But the philosophical understanding of mental realities—including thoughts, mental images, emotions, desires, dreams, and consciousness itself—had made no comparable progress. Scientists had found effective methods for "meditating on," or measuring, objective physical things, but philosophers had failed to devise methods for rigorously observing subjective mental events.

William James (1842–1910), the great American pioneer of psychology, felt that the scientific understanding of the mind in his day was hardly more developed than physics before Galileo.[7] Since 1600, he noted, scientists had devised methods for investigating the external world that could be subjected to mathematical analysis. In this way, questions that had long been argued over by philosophers were finally solved by the empirical methods of science. The more science progressed, the fewer problems remained in the hands of philosophers.[8]

The career of William James provides numerous examples that, if followed seriously, might have led Western psychology to a more complete and balanced understanding of the mind than we have today. After being educated as a youth in the United States and Europe, in 1861 James enrolled in the Laurence Scientific School at Harvard, and three years later he entered Harvard Medical School, from which he graduated in 1869. In part due to the biological determinism in which he was indoctrinated during his medical studies, he began to experience repeated bouts of severe depression, which he later described as a descent into a profound crisis—of spirituality, of being, of meaning, and of will. But in 1870, he had a revelation that free will was no illusion after all and that he could use his will to lift himself from his depression. He decided that he was not simply an automaton ruled by biological processes in his body, and he made his first act of free will to believe in free will.

James began teaching anatomy and physiology at Harvard in 1873, and two years later he began teaching psychology and established there the first laboratory for the scientific study of the mind. He defined psychology as "the Science of Mental Life, both of its phenomena and their conditions. The phenomena are such things as we call feelings, desires, cognitions, reasonings, decisions, and the like."[9] While physicists studied physical things that were accessible to all competent observers, psychologists were to examine subjectively experienced mental processes and their relations to their objects, to the brain, and to the rest of the world. But mental experiences are private and inaccessible to direct observation by the tools of science. So James proposed that psychology should primarily use introspection to study mental processes.[10] But the direct observation of one's own mental states and processes, he argued, must be complemented with comparative research, such as the study of animal behavior, and experimental brain science.

While James focused on the introspective observation of *conscious* mental experience, the Austrian neurologist Sigmund Freud (1856–1939) became well known for his theories of the *unconscious* mind. His pioneering work was crucial to the creation of the psychoanalytic school of psychology, in which the therapist seeks to discover connections among the unconscious components of patients' mental processes. On the basis of patients' verbal reports of their subjective experiences while awake and while dreaming, Freud sought to fathom the hidden mechanisms of the mind.

By the early twentieth century, neither academic psychologists nor psychoanalysts had succeeded in devising rigorous means of observing mental processes firsthand. So after only thirty years, introspection was largely abandoned as a means for scientifically investigating the mind. There were two major reasons for this.[11] One was that researchers working in different laboratories had a difficult time replicating each other's findings, for their subjects who practiced introspection tended to "observe" what the researchers expected them to experience. Note that the psychologists made no significant progress in refining their own introspection, and they didn't practice it much, at least in their professional capacity. Rather, they had their experimental subjects examine their own minds, but with no sustained, rigorous training that would enable them to make accurate, reliable observations. So even though the scientists explicitly used introspection in their research, they left it in the hands of amateurs. Introspection was never developed beyond the level of "folk psychology."

The second major reason introspection was rejected by the scientific community was that it went against the grain of scientific research over the previous three hundred years, which had consistently focused on objective, physical, quantitative realities. By the opening decades of the twentieth century, the natural sciences had proven so successful—especially when compared to religion and philosophy—that a growing number of people equated the natural world with the physical world. In other words, the only things they considered to be real were the things scientists could measure: namely, physical entities and processes. Anything else was deemed "supernatural," and therefore nonexistent, or at least irrelevant to scientific inquiry.

With the rejection of the scientific use of introspection, academic psychology in the English-speaking world shifted to behaviorism, which did all it could to eliminate references to subjectively experienced mental states and processes.[12] John B. Watson (1878–1958), one of the pioneers of American behaviorism, declared that psychology was no longer to be the science of mental life, as William James had defined it. As "a purely objective experimental branch of natural science," he said it should "never use the terms consciousness, mental states, mind, content, introspectively verifiable, imagery, and the like."[13] This taboo against subjective experience was motivated in part by the association of the mind (or soul) with religion and in part by the apparently nonphysical nature of mental events.[14] Scientists' suspicion of anything religious is quite understandable, for to them, religion required unquestioning belief in authority. Science, in contrast, placed the highest priority on experiential knowledge.

Here was the rub. For experiential evidence to be regarded as empirical evidence, it had to be verifiable—accessible to multiple competent observers. But mental processes can be observed only internally. They cannot be detected by any outside observer or by any of the instruments of science, which are designed to measure all known kinds of physical realities. Consequently, psychologists found themselves in a quandary: should they continue in the spirit of empiricism, which had been at the root of scientific progress for the last three hundred years? Or should they stick to the observation of external, physical objects, the domain of reality where science had enjoyed so much progress since the time of Galileo? They opted for the latter, narrower focus. Behaviorists chose to study human behavior and not any mysterious inner, spiritual, mental entities, which seemed to have no physical properties of their own.[15]

Behaviorism, at least as it developed in academic research psychology, was primarily concerned with finding effective ways of understanding the human mind through behavior, rather than drawing conclusions about the real nature of mental processes. This was like trying to understand human anatomy and physiology without ever performing autopsies—which was prohibited in medieval medicine. Most of the behaviorists were well aware of their mental states, but they thought psychology would develop faster and with fewer digressions if it left introspection out for a while. However, more radical behaviorists, beginning with Watson, took the further step of declaring that mental processes in general and consciousness in particular did not exist at all—precisely because they had no physical attributes![16] This was a clear case of denial, in which an ideological commitment to materialism nullified experiential evidence that didn't accord with that belief system. But even worse, behaviorists equated behavior with psychological processes themselves. Robots exhibit behavior, but they aren't conscious and have no subjective experiences. Humans also exhibit behavior, but however scrupulously you examine it, physical behavior by itself provides no evidence even for the existence of the mental realities that we all experience. The claim that subjective experience can be reduced to objective behavior is nothing short of intellectual dishonesty or else profound confusion.

By 1960, the limitations of ignoring mental processes were becoming increasingly apparent to academic psychologists. The new field of cognitive psychology began to take subjective experience more seriously, and since the rise of cognitive neuroscience in the closing decades of the twentieth century, a great deal of attention has been given to the brain processes related to subjective experience. Great progress has been made in identifying specific parts and functions of the brain that are necessary for vision and the other physical senses and for specific mental processes such as memory, emotion, and imagination. This is a perfectly legitimate way of investigating mental experience indirectly, for it draws on the strengths of four hundred years of scientific research into physical realities. But the actual nature of mental processes themselves remains as mysterious as ever.

What is the relationship between mental and brain processes—between our subjective experiences and our physical "hardware"? Is it purely *causal*, with brain processes generating subjective experience? Or are mental and neural processes really the same thing, viewed from inside and outside? Christof Koch, who works at the cutting edge of research on the neural correlates of consciousness, comments on this question: "The characters of brain states and of phenomenal states appear too different to be completely reducible to each other. I suspect that the relationship is more complex than traditionally envisioned. For now, it is best to keep an open mind on this matter and to concentrate on identifying the correlates of consciousness in the brain."[17] As a professionally trained neuroscientist, naturally he draws on his strengths, namely studying the brain. But nothing has been learned about the actual nature of subjective experience by studying the brain alone. When we objectively observe brain states, they exhibit none of the characteristics of mental states, and when we subjectively observe mental states, they display none of the characteristics of brain activity.

Many neuroscientists believe that mental processes originate in the brain as emergent properties. An emergent property arises from a large configuration of components, but is not present in any one of those parts individually. For example, a single H_2O molecule at room temperature is not fluid. But a large body of water molecules exhibits the quality of fluidity. Fluidity is a well-understood physical quality that is easily measured with the instruments of technology. Likewise, many emergent properties of physical entities are themselves physical and can be measured, such as blood flow and electrical and chemical changes within the brain. Mental processes, in contrast, bear no physical qualities and cannot be objectively measured in any way. Since they are radically unlike any other emergent properties that arise in the physical world, there seems to be little justification for regarding them as emergent properties of any physical entity.

Some neuroscientists, however, gloss over these problems and perhaps inadvertently cloud the issue by simply declaring that mental processes are the same as their neural bases.[18] This is a plausible hypothesis, but it has never been demonstrated scientifically. So it is intellectually dishonest to claim this as a scientific conclusion; at present it is nothing more than an unverified opinion. Here there is a danger of genuine science degenerating into pseudo-science. One of the characteristics of pseudo-science is that it tries to prove *that* a hypothesis is true, rather than investigating *whether* it is true. The assumption that the hypothesis is true and only needs proving replaces the open-mindedness that typifies the scientific method. Thus, many neuroscientists have adopted exactly this pseudo-scientific approach in trying to prove *that,* not *whether* subjective experiences can be fully comprehended in terms of physical processes within the brain.[19] Recall that in seventeenth-century Europe, the soul was widely believed to have both supernatural and natural attributes. In their insistence on understanding the human mind as a purely *natural* entity, scientists have treated it as if it must be *physical,* even though it displays no physical attributes and can't be detected with any physical instrument. This is a central problem for the entire scientific study of the mind, which has yet to be resolved.

Psychologists continue to study the mind indirectly by questioning conscious subjects and observing their behavior. In this way they directly investigate the physical *effects* of mental processes. And neuroscientists study the mind indirectly by exploring the neural bases of subjective experience. In these ways they directly investigate the physical *correlates* of mental events, which may be either *causes* or *effects.* The combined disciplines of psychology and neuroscience are now known as cognitive science. If researchers in this field confined their inquiries to the study of behavior and the brain alone, they would have no idea that subjective experience even exists. The only way experimenters can be certain that mental states exist is to experience them for themselves. This brings home the value of William James's insistence that introspection be fully incorporated into the scientific study of the mind.

Cognitive scientists have never devised any sophisticated means for examining mental events themselves. Such observations they leave to paid subjects (usually undergraduate students) who have no professional training in observing or reporting on mental processes. By leaving introspection in the hands of amateurs, scientists guarantee that the direct observation of the mind remains at the level of folk psychology. In this regard, let's place cognitive science in the context of the other natural sciences. Experimental physicists are professionally trained to observe physical processes, and biologists are professionally trained to observe biological processes. *Cognitive scientists have taken on the challenge of understanding mental processes, but unlike all other natural scientists, they receive no professional training in observing the realities that comprise their field of inquiry.*

This is not to say that the cognitive sciences haven't learned much about the mind. In fact, psychologists and neuroscientists have learned a great deal about a wide range of mental processes (some of them inaccessible to introspection) and their corresponding brain states. And there have been many valuable applications of their knowledge in diagnosing and treating mental diseases. Neuroscientists have substituted objective measurements of the brain for meditations on their corresponding subjective mental processes. This approach has yielded great insights into the neural bases of the mind, but very little understanding of the actual nature and origins of consciousness and all other subjective mental processes.

Over the past century, the failure of cognitive scientists to devise any rigorous means of directly observing mental realities has led to their similar conclusion that introspection cannot be used as a scientific method of inquiry. This belief, which continues to be widely held by psychologists and neuroscientists, still allows for exploring the mind by way of behavior and brain activity. But it undermines the value of introspection, and implicitly supports the assumption that mental processes are really nothing more than brain processes viewed from a subjective perspective. The implication is that brain processes are real, but mental processes are illusory.

But now, with the ease of global transportation and communication, we have much greater access to all the world's civilizations than ever before. Consequently, a rapidly growing number of cognitive scientists are now showing keen personal and professional interest in previously unknown contemplative traditions, along with those developed in the West. Therefore, the centuries-long scientific rejection of meditation may soon be a thing of the past.

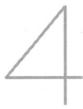

SCIENTIFIC STUDIES OF MEDITATION

Are our mental states and behavior entirely determined by such physical influences as brain activity and genes, or can we improve our sense of well-being through our own efforts, including meditation? This is a fundamental question that underlies all scientific studies of meditation. Recall that William James fell into deep, suicidal depression partly in response to the belief—which was prevalent in the mid-nineteenth century—that humans are mere puppets jerked around by biochemical processes in our bodies. He pulled himself out of the rut by recognizing that the scientific evidence supporting that reductionistic hypothesis was not conclusive. Research over the past few years has made this robotic view of human nature even more dubious.

One of the most fascinating fields of neuroscientific inquiry nowadays concerns neuroplasticity, or the ability of neurons in the brain to change in response to experience. What this implies for us in our daily lives is that we can actually change our brains by altering our thoughts, attitudes, and behavior. Research points to the brain as a continuously changing organ that responds structurally not only to the demands of the external environment but also to internally generated states, including aspects of consciousness. In one pioneering experiment, neuroscientists at Harvard Medical School had one group of volunteers practice a piano exercise every day for one week, while another group merely imagined that they were doing the exercise, moving their fingers and playing the notes only in their minds. At the end of the week, the motor cortex, which is the region of the brain that controls finger movements, had become larger in the actual players, which was the expected result—but the same change had also occurred in the brains of the virtual players! Merely imagining that they had been playing the piano had led to measurable physical changes in the brain. So much for the old saying, "It's not real, it's only in your mind!"

Researchers at the Salk Institute for Biological Studies in La Jolla, California have shown that the adult brain can change its structure, its connections, and therefore its functions—a capacity for change that scientists had long believed was lost in early childhood. This means that we can voluntarily transform our minds and brains throughout our lifetime by choosing our environment, our way of life, and the types of mental activity we engage in. One way that neuroplasticity occurs is through neurogenesis, or the generation of new brain cells and, more importantly, new connections of synapses. A healthy human brain contains about 100 billion nerve cells, or neurons. Each neuron has long filamentary projections called axons and dendrites, which transmit information in the form of electrical pulses. Dendrites carry signals into the neurons, and axons carry signals to other cells. The junction between an axon and a dendrite is called a synapse, and information is carried across synapses by chemical messengers called neurotransmitters. Neurogenesis increases the connections among synapses, and this, more than the generation of new brain cells alone, has a real impact on the way our minds work.

Neurogenesis enables us to make new connections to recognize novelty; otherwise, our previous fixed connections can cause us to see even new things in an old, stale way. This ability to create new connections generally declines with age, but it can be enhanced by living in an "enriched environment," in which we encounter interesting, new, and challenging things to do and experience. This enriched environment can also include the world of our imagination and all the activities we do with our minds. Therefore, meditation may be one of the most effective ways of rejuvenating our brains and minds.

Recent discoveries by scientists at McGill University in Montreal challenge the view that human beings are slaves to their genes, their neurotransmitters, and their brain wiring. The new field these researchers are exploring is epigenetics, the study of functional changes in the genome that do not involve alterations in the DNA sequencing of the genes themselves. Genes may be very active, somewhat active, or dormant. The extent of their activity is determined by their chemical environment, and that's influenced by, among other things, parental care. Environmental factors can lead to the production of proteins called transcription factors, which determine how genes influence the rest of the human organism. The gene is made up of two segments: one produces proteins, and the second is a regulatory site that turns the gene on and off. Transcription factors interact with the latter. Studies of animals and humans have shown that nurturing caregivers and low levels of stress are important in producing appropriate levels of the brain chemicals that are necessary for emotional health and balance.[1] The genes we inherit from our ancestors, influenced by millions of years of natural selection, do not inevitably determine our personalities, abilities, or character. On the contrary, our physical and mental behavior may influence whether our genes will be very active, somewhat active, or dormant. For example, a child may have a genetic predisposition for attention deficit/hyperactivity disorder (ADHD), but with attentional training, the activity of the relevant genes can be reduced or stopped.

Stress impairs neurogenesis, but certain kinds of activities promote it, and this is where meditation may play a key role. Until recently, most scientific studies of meditation were considered to be "fringe science." However, this field began to draw public attention in the late 1960s when doctors from Harvard Medical School and the University of California at Irvine found that a group practicing Transcendental Meditation (TM) showed a decrease in stress and anxiety, related to lower oxygen consumption and a slower breathing rate. Such meditation involves concentrating for twenty minutes or longer on a mentally recited mantra with the aim of transcending the normal state of consciousness. The researchers theorized that two activities—repetition, as in the recitation of a word or prayer, and deliberately disregarding competing thoughts—led to a "relaxation response."[2] As a result of similar studies over several decades, meditation of this sort is now a recommended treatment for hypertension, cardiac arrhythmias, chronic pain, insomnia, and the side effects of cancer and AIDS therapy.[3]

Meditation is becoming widely popular as an adjunct to conventional medical therapies for the treatment of a wide variety of chronic illnesses, including cancer, hypertension, and psoriasis.[4] Researchers at the Yale School of Medicine have recently been studying the effects of meditation for improving the quality of life of patients who are dying with AIDS. They have recognized that even in cases of terminal illness, quality of life remains important, as does the quality and peacefulness of a person's death. At the California Pacific Medical Center in San Francisco, the Zen Hospice Project (ZHP) has been designed to learn how being with dying hospice residents affects hospice volunteers' well-being and to understand the role of spiritual practice in alleviating the fear of death. In this project a forty-hour training program has been offered to beginning hospice volunteers with an emphasis on compassion, equanimity, mindfulness, and practical bedside care. The effects of this training have been found to include a heightened sense of compassion and a decreased fear of death.

In a related study, researchers confirmed the beneficial effects of regular mindfulness meditation among caregivers at a Zen hospice.[5] Mindfulness, in this context, is understood as a state in which one is acutely aware of and focused on the reality of the present moment, accepting and acknowledging it, without getting caught up in thoughts about or emotional reactions to the situation.[6] In mindfulness meditation the hospice caregivers were taught to place their awareness on their breathing and notice as thoughts, emotions, and sensations arose and passed away. When they became aware of being lost in the contents of their mind—thoughts, emotions, and internal mental chatter—they were encouraged to redirect their attention gently to the breath until their awareness was stabilized.

Over time, participants in this study found they could more easily bring their attention back to the moment. By practicing meditation in action, throughout the day they attended to what they were doing and why. Mindfulness was experienced as not holding onto the past, the future, or "now-ness," but relaxing into the immediacy of whatever was happening. As a way of training the mind, they applied mindfulness to their everyday activities of service: cooking for, washing, feeding, sitting with, and listening to residents. Benefits they experienced as a result of this practice included a sense of inseparability between caregivers and residents, finding stillness while engaged in activities, letting go of wishing things were otherwise and fearing what might be, and maintaining clear mindfulness in the midst of emotions.

Beginning in the late 1970s, Jon Kabat-Zinn, a researcher at the Stress Reduction Clinic at the University of Massachusetts Medical Center, developed a Mindfulness-Based Stress Reduction (MBSR) program, which is now being taught in more than 250 clinics throughout the world. As Kabat-Zinn pointed out in a meeting in 1990 with the Dalai Lama on mindfulness, emotions, and health, stress aggravates the symptoms of all known illnesses, from the common cold to cancer.[7] So alleviating stress with meditation can potentially have an enormous impact on our physical and psychological well-being. For example, researchers at the University of Toronto have shown that meditation can prevent relapse of depression in patients with a history of recurrent mood disorder, and other studies support this finding.[8] A rapidly growing number of studies of meditation at major research universities worldwide are demonstrating its benefits for an ever-widening array of psychological and physical problems.[9] They have found that even brief periods of meditation throughout the day are more restful and healthy for the body and mind than taking naps.

In one such study, Kabat-Zinn teamed up with Richard Davidson, who heads the W. M. Keck Laboratory for Functional Brain Imaging at the University of Wisconsin at Madison. Davidson first began studying the relationship among emotions, the brain, and meditation in the 1970s. Kabat-Zinn and Davidson recently conducted a study of the effects of eight weeks of basic training in mindfulness meditation on a group of highly stressed workers for a Wisconsin biotech firm. Preliminary results demonstrate that those who received this training showed an increase in left-prefrontal lobe activation both at rest and when presented with emotional challenges. Increased activation of this area of the brain is associated with positive emotions and reduced stress, along with improvements in the immune system.[10]

Since then, Davidson and his team have studied highly advanced Tibetan Buddhist contemplatives who have engaged in meditative training for as long as 60,000 hours. When the researchers hooked up these monks to EEG sensors, they found a striking increase in gamma waves generated by the brain as a whole and heightened neural activity in the left prefrontal cortex, an area correlated with reported feelings of happiness. Although it is not entirely clear how one can interpret these data in terms of human experience, they do suggest that such mental training triggers integrative mechanisms in the brain and may induce short-term and long-term neural changes.[11]

Another study by researchers at Harvard University at Massachusetts General Hospital[12] suggests that long-term meditation may increase the thickness of the cortex, which is the outer layer of the brain. Using MRI measurements, they found that meditation involving focused attention to one's own mental states and processes led to a thickening of brain regions associated with attention, introspection, and sensory processing. Even forty minutes of daily meditation appears to thicken parts of the cerebral cortex involved in attention and sensory processing. Differences in prefrontal cortical thickness were most pronounced in the older participants, suggesting that meditation might offset age-related deterioration of attention and mindfulness of one's surroundings.[13]

Psychologists at the University of Oregon have been investigating the possibility of training young children to enhance executive attention—the ability to regulate our psychological and behavioral responses, particularly in conflict situations. When our emotions are strongly aroused, our capacity for executive attention enables us to stay focused on what is important and not get caught up in compulsive thoughts and memories. This aspect of attention undergoes particularly rapid development between two and seven years of age, but it is thought to continue to develop until early adulthood. In one recent study, children between the ages of four and six (the ideal group for studying such training effects) were given training designed to enhance executive attention.[14] This study showed for the first time that executive attention skills can be trained in young children, and could potentially lead to better types of treatment for children with attentional and other behavioral problems. The researchers also believe that the effect of attention training may extend to more general skills such as those measured by intelligence tests. In other words, increasing your attention skills may also help to increase your IQ.

One of the most important studies of the effects of meditation on attention was recently conducted by neuroscientist Amishi Jha and two of her colleagues at the University of Pennsylvania. They compared the effects of two groups of meditators engaged in two types of mindfulness training. The first consisted of novices to meditation who participated in an eight-week mindfulness-based stress reduction course, which entailed just thirty minutes each day of focusing on their breathing, gently bringing their attention back to the object whenever it strayed. A second group comprised experienced meditators participating in a one-month intensive mindfulness retreat, practicing ten to twelve hours each day. A third group consisted of people who had never meditated and received no training at all. At the conclusion of their respective training courses, it was found that the first group was better able to focus their attention on their meditative object than the second and third groups, while the second group was more competent than the first and third groups in becoming mindfully aware of their surroundings.[15]

While attention training is bound to be a key factor in bringing about positive psychological changes, other aspects of the mind, such as desires, attitudes, and emotions, also need to be taken into account.[16] In the fall of 2000, the Dalai Lama met with a group of cognitive psychologists to explore the theme of destructive emotions from scientific and Buddhist perspectives.[17] I had the privilege of serving as co-interpreter for this meeting. After several days of fascinating dialogue across disciplines and cultures, the Dalai Lama commented that as useful as such discussions were, it was most important that we apply our collective knowledge and experience to be of practical benefit in the world. One of the participants, Paul Ekman, a professor emeritus of psychology at the University of California at San Francisco, rose to this challenge and set into motion the development of the Cultivating Emotional Balance (CEB) program. Both he and the Dalai Lama asked me to join him in this research project from its inception. Paul and I put together an eight-week training program including psychological interventions and meditations drawn from the Buddhist tradition. This integrated training included practices for enhancing executive attention, mindfulness, and the cultivation of empathy, loving-kindness, and compassion. In 2003 we ran a pilot study, and since then, under the direction of Margaret Kemeny, another psychologist at UCSF, we have conducted two clinical trials in which we have offered this training to groups of schoolteachers. We recommended that all participants meditate at least twenty-five minutes per day, and they were also instructed on how to "season each day" with mindfulness, which involved interspersing moments of meditation throughout the day, for instance, while stopped at a stoplight, while waiting in line, in between reading e-mail messages, and so on.

We found that participation in the CEB training was associated with significant, and in many cases dramatic, reductions in depression, chronic anxiety, negative emotions (such as irritation, frustration, and hostility), and compulsive thinking. On the positive side, this training resulted in significant increases in positive emotions (such as patience, empathy, affection, and compassion), mindfulness, attentiveness to others, and more restful sleep. These psychological benefits were noted at the end of the training, and they were still present five months later.

In terms of the participants' nervous systems, as a result of this training they experienced less "wear and tear" when confronted with an emotionally distressing situation, and they returned to equilibrium more quickly once the episode was over. Hormonal responses also changed for the better. Cortisol, often referred to as the primary "stress hormone," is a steroid hormone produced in the adrenal gland in response to stress. It is needed to maintain normal physiological processes during times of stress, but excessively high levels of cortisol in the bloodstream can lead to impaired cognitive performance, suppressed thyroid function, blood sugar imbalances such as hyperglycemia, decrease in bone density and muscle tissue, and high blood pressure. Recent evidence suggests that excessively low levels of cortisol can be associated with depression and burnout, as well as risk for inflammatory diseases. Participants in the CEB training showed faster recovery from cortisol activity, which indicates that their cortisol systems may have been more adaptively responding to emotionally upsetting situations. In short, this training enhanced the ability of the schoolteachers to recover psychologically, autonomically, and hormonally from emotional upsets. Given the highly stressful nature of their profession, it seems likely that the mental training that helped them may help virtually everyone else who is trying to cope with the difficulties of modern life.

One of the most interesting aspects of the human psyche is what Ekman calls the refractory period. This generally follows immediately upon some emotionally disturbing experience, and he points out that for as long as it lasts, "our thinking cannot incorporate information that does not fit, maintain, or justify the emotion we are feeling," and this "biases the way we see the world and ourselves."[18] For example, if you have become angry with a colleague at work, during your refractory period you can focus your attention only on aspects of this person's personality and behavior that support your current feelings of hostility. Even when you bring to mind neutral or even positive behavior on his part, you are bound to view it in a negative light, and for the time being you may be blind to all his virtues.

With regard to the refractory period, meditation becomes a kind of "dashboard for your emotions," enabling you to check the gauges and objectively decide if you're about to overheat, so you're not caught by surprise when your mind begins to boil over. The neural basis of such emotional reactions is the limbic system, which is connected to the prefrontal cortex. By acting on the prefrontal cortex, meditation can help to restore our emotional balance when we become upset by fear or anger. For most of us, it is only a quarter of a second between the trigger event and the response of the amygdala, or fear center. In that fraction of a second, our emotions have time to swamp our judgment, and they often do.[19] Meditation—which brings increased sensitivity to such reactions—provides us with the opportunity to break this apparent chain reaction by allowing us to recognize "the spark before the flame." In that way we can begin to make more informed choices about which emotions to act on and which to let remain unexpressed.

Training in meditation may also be helpful in augmenting a wide array of other human virtues, including the simple quality of goodness. During the meeting with the Dalai Lama in 2000, Paul Ekman had the opportunity to spend a few minutes with him in one-to-one conversation. "He held my hands while we talked," he recalled, "and I was filled with a sense of goodness and a unique total body sensation that I have no words to describe." After struggling with anger and rage for most of his adult life, Ekman now says he understands what it actually feels like to be cheery and optimistic almost every day. At the age of seventy-two, he commented recently, "If I were thirty years younger, I'd take on as a scientific task to try to explain what happened that day." He is eager to know how the Dalai Lama cured him literally overnight of the explosive temper that had had him in psychoanalysis for years. With that aim in mind, he's recently interviewed eight others who have experienced similar transformations after meeting the Dalai Lama.[20]

I had my first private meeting with the Dalai Lama in the autumn of 1971, when I was living in Dharamsala, India. That first encounter had a deep impact on me, which was reinforced eight years later when I had the opportunity to serve as his interpreter for his lecture tour of Europe, just before his first visit to the United States. I found that being in his presence day after day was like dwelling in a field of kindness, which brought with it a sense of serenity and well-being that I'd never experienced before. Those of us who have encountered such extraordinary people are bound to ask: were they born that way, or can their exceptional qualities of wisdom and compassion be cultivated through training? In reflecting on his own life, the Dalai Lama has made it quite clear that his spiritual practice, including daily meditation for over fifty years, has deeply transformed his mind in many beneficial ways.[21] Each year he travels worldwide, teaching meditative practices that draw on 2,500 years of experience from the Buddhist tradition, as well as his own personal experience.

A rapidly growing number of cognitive scientists, especially ones who are just beginning their professional careers, are expressing an interest in combining the scientific methods of psychology and neuroscience with the contemplative approaches of Buddhism and other traditions. They wish to explore the mind from multiple perspectives. Since 2003, the Mind and Life Institute, which has sponsored meetings on Buddhism and science with the Dalai Lama since 1987, has been holding weeklong summer research institutes attended by graduate and postgraduate students in the mind sciences and humanities. During these intensive seminars, senior research scientists share the findings of their latest research on meditation, and Buddhist scholars and contemplatives teach Buddhist theory and meditation to all the participants. In this way, there is emerging a new generation of "contemplative scientists," people with professional training both in the cognitive sciences and in the theory and practice of meditation.

Along similar lines, in the winter of 2007, the Santa Barbara Institute for Consciousness Studies began holding a series of meditation retreats specifically for research scientists in the fields of psychology and neuroscience. For the past century, the mind sciences have sought to distance themselves from anything associated with religion or even philosophy. But now, scientists in this field are showing an unprecedented openness and curiosity to learn more about the physiological and psychological benefits of meditation and to explore its possible value for investigating the nature of the mind from within.

This could signal a major turning point in the history of science, which for its first 400 years fixed its attention solely on the objective, physical world. In the future, the unified focus of outwardly directed, objective scientific inquiry and inwardly directed contemplative inquiry is bound to bring an unprecedented depth to our understanding of the nature and potentials of consciousness.

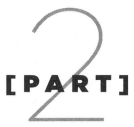

[PART]

MEDITATION IN THEORY AND PRACTICE

In my introduction to part I, I made the rather audacious claim that meditation is much more than a pleasant form of relaxation or a type of stress therapy—that through meditation one can unlock the deepest secrets of the self and its relation to the universe. Now, in part II, I will describe some of the enormous variety of meditative theories and their respective practices. We should not be surprised that meditation has been applied to so many areas of human inquiry and with such great subtlety. After all, Western science has been in existence for only four centuries, but meditation has been around for at least four millennia. Although it originated in ancient civilizations that did not have the printing press, there is an enormous literature on contemplation, often supporting an oral tradition that has been handed down for more than a hundred generations.

Since for most readers this is new material, I will present it gradually—but not by merely describing these meditative forms. You will come to a much deeper understanding, and perhaps find some relevance in meditation for your own life, if you put some effort into trying the practices that precede each theoretical discussion. Of course, these techniques require effort and dedication to bear fruit. In that, they are no different than any other skill one would develop and master. Nevertheless, I believe that engaging with these practices—even briefly—will at least provide a hint of their depth and potential.

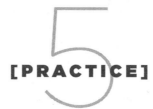

[PRACTICE]

ATTENDING TO THE BREATH OF LIFE

Find a quiet room where you can sit alone without being disturbed. Soften the lighting and find a comfortable place to sit for twenty-five minutes—on a chair or, if you're comfortable, sitting cross-legged on a cushion. You can also lie on your back on your bed, for instance, with your head resting on a pillow, your legs straight, your arms out to the sides, palms up, and your eyes either shut or partly open. Whatever your position, see that your back is straight and that you feel physically at ease.

Now focus your attention on your body, experiencing the sensations from the soles of your feet up to the top of your head, both within your body and on its surfaces. Be totally present in your body, and if you note any areas that feel tight, breathe into them (at least in your imagination), and as you exhale, breathe out that tension. Be aware of the sensations in the muscles of your face—your jaws, mouth, and forehead—and relax them, letting your face be as relaxed as a baby's when it's fast asleep. Especially be aware of your eyes. The poets tell us the eyes are windows of the soul. When we're upset, the eyes tend to feel hard and piercing, as if they're bulging from their sockets. Not only do our mental states influence our eyes, but we can also influence our minds by softening the eyes. Let them be soft and relaxed, with no contraction between the eyebrows or in the forehead. Set your whole body at ease.

For the duration of these twenty-five minutes, apart from the natural movement of respiration, let your body be as still as possible. This will help to stabilize your mind and enable you to focus your attention with greater continuity. If you're sitting on a chair or cross-legged, slightly raise your sternum and keep your abdominal muscles soft and relaxed, so that when you breathe in, you feel the sensations of the breath go right down to your belly. If your breath is shallow, you'll feel just the abdomen expand. If you inhale more deeply, first the abdomen, then the diaphragm will expand. And if you take a very deep breath, first the belly, then the diaphragm, and finally the chest will expand. Try taking three slow, deep breaths, feeling the sensations of respiration throughout your body, inhaling almost to full capacity, then releasing the breath effortlessly.

Then return to normal, unforced respiration, mindfully attending to the sensations of the breath wherever they arise in the body. Breathe as effortlessly as possible, as if you were deeply asleep. And with each exhalation, think of releasing excess tension in your body, and let go of any clinging to involuntary thoughts that have arisen in your mind. Continue relaxing all the way through the end of the out-breath until the in-breath flows in spontaneously like the tide.

As you attend to the gentle rhythm of your respiration, you may hear your neighbor's dog barking, the sounds of traffic, or the voices of other people. Take note of whatever arises to your five physical senses, moment by moment, and let it be. Notice also what goes on in your mind, including thoughts and emotions that arise in response to stimuli from your environment. Each time your attention gets caught up in sensory stimuli or thoughts and memories, breathe out, release your mind from these preoccupations, and gently return to your breath. Let your attention remain within the field of sensations of your body, and let the world and the activities of your mind flow around you unimpeded, without trying to control or influence them in any way.

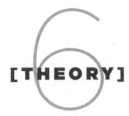

[THEORY]

COMING TO OUR SENSES

One of the most persistent of all delusions is the conviction that the source of our dissatisfaction lies outside ourselves. No matter who we are, we think the world is in such miserable shape because of the behavior of people who aren't like us. Political liberals are certain that conservatives are to blame for the world's problems, while the conservatives are just as convinced that they are part of the solution. Political activists blame the politically apathetic for not taking responsibility for their government's policies, while the general public blames their government for their misfortunes and regards their financial contributions to the governance of their homeland as a "tax burden." Religious believers find fault with people who belong to other sects within their own religion, as well as followers of other religions and nonbelievers. And atheists, tenaciously clinging to their own materialistic creed, attribute the world's evils to religious believers. Each of us is convinced that God, or at least truth and righteousness, is on our side.

This ubiquitous delusion is just as prevalent on the local level as on an international scale. If we find problems in our home cities or neighborhoods, we believe that other people are to blame. About half of marriages in the United States end in divorce, and in most cases each partner will say the other person is at fault. Even when we acknowledge that our own conduct hasn't been entirely perfect, we easily conclude that the other person drove us to it. If only *they* had behaved better in the first place, *we* wouldn't have strayed! The same is true when there's strife between parents and their children—it's always someone else at the root of the problem.

Here is a hypothetical solution, and I invite you to image how it might work. Close your eyes and imagine that everyone else on Earth who is contributing to the world's misery is suddenly transported to the Moon. In ancient India some people thought that the souls of those who had not achieved liberation from the cycle of rebirth transmigrated to the Moon, where they were greeted by their ancestors. So there's an old precedent for this idea. As you envision this cleansing of the home planet of all evildoers, make sure you don't leave any of them out. When you've finished, open your eyes and look around you.

Welcome to the looney bin! While you've been sending all the people on your blacklist to the Moon, you can be sure that someone else has done the same to you. We've now transported all 6.5 billion people from the Earth to the Moon. And if you look through a telescope back to Earth, you may see all nonhuman species throwing a global party—thank goodness their homeland is finally free of the cancerous blight known as the human race! Without our interference, the ecosphere swiftly begins to recover its balance and looks more and more like a Garden of Eden. And the Moon looks like an immensely overpopulated, barren, and bleak penal colony. As the philosopher Jean-Paul Sartre said, famously: "Hell is other people."

We all tend to think that other people are the problem and that we're part of the solution. But this just doesn't add up. There's no question that others do things that contribute to the world's misery and pain, and it would be great if they saw the error of their ways. But let's not hold our breath, waiting for them to shape up. At least in our own little corners of the world, we can start to take responsibility for our own behavior—to create a better future for ourselves and for those who are closest to us.

We can start by restoring balance to our own bodies and minds, and the preceding practice of mindfulness of breathing can be a big step in that direction. When the human race stops upsetting the balance of nature due to our greed and delusion, the ecosphere heals itself. Soil regains its fertility, bodies of water purify themselves, the problem of global warming resolves itself, the atmosphere becomes free of all kinds of pollutants, and the ozone layer restores itself. At the micro level, each of us disrupts the balance of our body-minds whenever we succumb to emotional upsets driven by insecurity, fear, craving, hostility, or stupidity. Such emotional turbulence adversely affects our brains, our immune system, our hormones, and the nervous system as a whole. As we bring mindful attention to the rhythm of our respiration, we can see how disturbing thoughts and emotions disrupt and constrict our breathing, and this in turn throws the rest of the body out of balance. Our personal ecology goes out of whack.

The result of such body-mind imbalance is the feeling of being physically and emotionally stressed out—we bounce back and forth between psychological hyperactivity and exhaustion. These symptoms are messages our afflicted bodies are sending us, but we often react by resorting to drugs, alcohol, work, entertainment, food, sleep, and a thousand other ways to numb the pain. We don't like the messages received from our bodies, so we muzzle the messengers.

Mindfulness of breathing is no cure-all, but it does bring us in touch with the local reality of our own respiration. The breath is our most constant source of sustenance—the body's ongoing ebb and flow with its natural environment—and when we upset its rhythm, we impede this supply line. But by mindfully, passively attending to the breath, we can gradually restore the rate and volume of the respiration that the body needs in each moment, and our vitality will return. This happens naturally when we get a good night's sleep, as the respiration flows without interference from disturbing thoughts and emotions. Conversely, when we experience a restless night punctuated with unpleasant dreams, we tend to feel exhausted in the morning. Our respiration has had little chance to restore balance to our body and mind. With training, we can learn to settle our breathing in its natural rhythm during the waking state, and experience far less physical and mental wear and tear.

The most ancient Indian literature on contemplation suggests that the earliest of all meditative practices was to focus one's attention on the sacred syllable "Om" together with the breath. Mindfulness of breathing was already well known at the time of the Buddha, and according to his own account, his enlightenment took place while he was engaging in such practice. His instructions were simple. Without deliberately controlling or modifying the breath in any way, begin by simply noting the length of each inhalation and exhalation. As your mind begins to calm, the volume of your respiration gradually subsides, and you will note that the in-breath and out-breath become relatively short. As time passes, you engage your attention more and more continuously with the breath throughout the entire inhalation and exhalation. Eventually, the rhythm of the breath becomes calmer and calmer, as your whole body is soothed.

Since the Buddha began teaching this practice, a hundred generations of Buddhist contemplatives throughout Asia have rediscovered its benefits for yielding not only inner calm and equanimity but also an inner sense of bliss. As this practice is developed and cultivated, negative emotions arise far less frequently, and when they do, they tend to subside without disturbing the mind as much as they did in the past. These results imply that the mind has an extraordinary capacity to heal itself when given a chance. Just as a wound heals when it is kept clean and a broken bone fuses together when it is well set, so can our psychological wounds heal when the attention is firmly settled on the breath, without straying into thoughts of craving or hostility.

In order to help stabilize the attention on the respiration and decrease wandering thoughts, many Buddhist meditators mentally count breaths. Others seek the same end by reciting the two syllables "buddho" (a variation of the word "buddha") with each in- and out-breath. And in the Tibetan Buddhist tradition a common practice is to recite the three syllables "Om Ah Hum" (pronounced "ohm-ah-hoong"), one syllable each during the inhalation, the pause at the end of the in-breath, and the exhalation. "Om" symbolizes the body, "Ah" symbolizes the speech, and "Hum" symbolizes the mind. The mental recitation of these syllables throughout respiration is believed to purify the body, speech, and mind. All of these techniques are adaptations of the original instructions by the Buddha on balancing and soothing the body and mind with mindfulness of breathing.

The breath also holds a central place in Jewish and Christian thought, beginning with the Book of Genesis, which states that God formed man from the dust of the ground and breathed into his nostrils the breath of life (Genesis 2:7). In the New Testament, the breath of Jesus is said to have a divine quality about it, for as Jesus breathes on his apostles, he says, "Receive the Holy Spirit" (John 20:22). The Greek monk and theologian Maximus the Confessor (580–662) simply declared, "God is breath."[1]

Meditation on the breath has been important to Christians beginning as early as the fourth century. Evagrius of Pontus reputedly approached the famous monk and hermit Macarius the Elder (300–391) and asked him for a word to live by. Macarius responded that he should secure the anchor rope of his mind to the rock of Jesus Christ and should repeat the "Jesus prayer" with each breath: "Lord Jesus, have mercy on me." This may be the first record of the recitation of the Jesus prayer in conjunction with mindfulness of breathing.[2]

This practice was further developed within the Greek Orthodox contemplative tradition during the medieval era. For example, Saint Symeon the

New Theologian (949–1022) taught a method of mindfulness of breathing in which the breath is gently controlled so that it gradually slows down, which helps to calm the mind.[3] The Greek contemplative Saint Gregory Palamas (1296–1359) also encouraged novice meditators to focus their awareness inward with the aid of the breath. He elaborated on this theme as follows:

> Since the intellect of those recently embarked on the spiritual path continually darts away again as soon as it has been concentrated, they must continually bring it back once more; for in their inexperience they are unaware that of all things it is the most difficult to observe and the most mobile. That is why some teachers recommend them to pay attention to the exhalation and inhalation of their breath, and to restrain it a little, so that while they are watching it the intellect, too, may be held in check.[4]

According to Saint Gregory, mindfulness of breathing, especially when combined with physical and mental stillness, naturally results in the slowing of the breath, and he called the culmination of this process "unified concentration." Those who become adept in this practice, he said, "strip their soul's powers free from every transient, fleeting and compound form of knowledge, from every type of sense-perception and, in general, from every bodily act that is under our sway, and, so far as they can, even from those not entirely under our sway, such as breathing."[5] In other words, deeply concentrating the mind with this practice draws our awareness inward, disengaging it from all kinds of bodily activity, from sensory experience of our surroundings, and even from thoughts. This is a time for peering deeply within our own being, rather than staying on the surface, keeping busy just for the sake of keeping busy.

The deeply spiritual implications of this practice were pointed out by the renowned Spanish contemplative Saint John of the Cross (1542–91), who wrote, "The soul that is united and transformed in God breathes God in God with the same divine breathing with which God, while in her, breathes her in himself."[6] These words express the intimate presence of God within each human being by way of the breath, a theme that appears in very early Christian theology. The deepest purpose of the Christian practice of mindfulness of breathing, then, is to make us aware of the dynamic presence of God within our own being.

Beginning a meditative practice is like planting a tiny sapling. Whether it takes deep root, grows to its full height, and remains healthy for many years depends on the type of soil it's planted in and the nourishment it gets. Our way of viewing reality, our values and priorities, and our way of life are the soil supporting our meditation. If these are conducive and supportive, meditation will flourish over the long term and can immensely enrich our lives. If not, our venture into meditation will most likely be brief, or at best sporadic and superficial.

Meditation in the early Christian tradition was strongly supported by the biblical statement that humans are created in the *image* of God (Genesis 1:27), and Christian contemplatives have long devoted themselves to their practice in order to live in the *likeness* of God, that is, to emulate his perfection to the best of their abilities. As for the highest of all Christian values, when Jesus was asked what was the greatest commandment, he responded, "'Love the Lord your God with all your heart and with all your soul and with all your mind.' This is the first and greatest commandment. And the second is like it: 'Love your neighbor as yourself. All the Law and the Prophets hang on these two commandments'" (Matthew 22:37–40).

In early Christianity, the *love* of God meant the heartfelt yearning to *know* God, characterized as the "changeless light," and only with such experiential insight into this ultimate reality could one find genuine happiness. Knowledge of God was believed to yield a "truth-given joy," which in turn led to "the perfect life." So at the deepest level, the only thing we really need to know is: how can we find this truth that will make us happy?

Although the earliest ideal of Buddhism was to escape the cycle of rebirth, around the beginning of the Christian era, a new Buddhist movement arose in India known as the Mahayana, or the "Great Vehicle." Advocates of this tradition found the goal of individual liberation too limited, and they promoted the "bodhisattva ideal" of striving for the highest possible state of spiritual awakening in order to liberate all beings from suffering and to bring each one to a lasting state of timeless joy. For countless lifetimes prior to his enlightenment, Gautama (later known as Buddha) led the life of a bodhisattva, setting the example for all who came after him. The fundamental premise underlying the bodhisattva way of life is that all beings have the potential to achieve the perfection of enlightenment, and it is our challenge to realize that potential in our daily lives. Only by thoroughly integrating the ideals of genuine happiness, truth, and virtue can we fully discover the meaning of life.

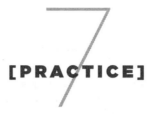

[PRACTICE]

THE UNION OF STILLNESS AND MOTION

Rest your body in a comfortable posture, whether sitting in a chair, sitting cross-legged, or lying on your back. Begin by "settling your body in its natural state,"[1] so that it is imbued with three qualities. The first quality is a physical sense of relaxation, ease, and comfort, which should persist throughout this entire twenty-five-minute session. The meditative practice itself is challenging enough, so it's important that you don't put yourself through any undue physical discomfort. Second, let your body be as still as possible, avoiding any unnecessary movement, such as fidgeting and scratching. Move only if your legs or back start to ache. Third, assume a posture of vigilance. If you are sitting upright, keep your back straight and slightly raise your sternum so that you can effortlessly breathe into your abdomen. If you are lying on your back, straighten your body, with your arms stretched out about thirty degrees from your torso. Let your eyes be partly open, but let your gaze be vacant.

Now "settle your speech in its natural state," which is effortless silence, and at the same time settle your respiration in its natural rhythm, as you did in the first meditation. With each exhalation, release any residual tightness in your body and continue relaxing and letting go all the way through the out-breath, until the in-breath flows in naturally and spontaneously. Breathe as effortlessly as if you were deeply asleep, but be clearly mindful of the sensations of the respiration throughout your body through the full course of the breathing cycle. At this point, as a preliminary exercise, for a few minutes you may deliberately calm your mind by counting your breaths, with one brief count at the very end of each inhalation. Alternatively, you may mentally recite "Jesus," the short version of the Jesus prayer, or the three syllables "Om Ah Hum" with each breath.

During the in-breath attend closely to the sensations of respiration wherever they arise in your body, and during the out-breath release any involuntary thoughts that may have arisen. Just let them go, as if they were leaves blown away by the breeze of your exhalation. Likewise, if your attention is caught by visual impressions or sounds from your environment, let them go, without trying to suppress them, and return your attention to the field of sensations within your body. You may count twenty-one breaths to help stabilize your mind.

Now proceed to the main practice for this session, which is called "settling the mind in its natural state." In the preliminary stage you withdrew your attention from your surroundings and practiced mindfulness of breathing within the field of your body. Now withdraw your attention from your body into the field of your mind, where you experience mental images, thoughts, emotions, desires, memories, and fantasies. You will still experience visual impressions, sounds, and tactile sensations, but focus your interest and attention on the mind alone. To help you identify this domain of experience, deliberately generate a mental image, which may be mundane, such as an apple or an orange, or sacred, like Jesus or Buddha. Focus your attention on that image until it vanishes. You have now placed your attention in the domain of the mind. Keep it there and wait for the next mental image to arise of its own accord. As soon as it appears, simply be aware of it, without grasping onto it or pushing it away.

Engaging in this practice is like occupying a front-row seat in the theater of your mind. You are not the director, trying to control who appears on the stage or what they do there. Nor are you an actor who gets up there and takes on various roles. You are a keen observer, but you watch passively without interacting with the things, people, and events that occur onstage. And you never know what's coming up next. When you first do this practice, you may find that your mind suddenly goes blank. Be patient and continue watching. After a while, images are bound to arise, and when they do, simply observe them without getting caught up in them or identifying with them. Simply be present with them, observing their every move, noting how they first arise, how they move and change over time, and how they eventually vanish.

Be aware too of discursive thoughts, or mental chitchat. You may begin by deliberately generating an ordinary thought, such as "this is the mind," or by mentally reciting a mantra or prayer such as the Jesus prayer. As that thought arises, observe it closely and note how it vanishes, whether all of a sudden or by gradually fading out. As soon as it's gone, keep your attention focused right where it was, for you are now observing the space of the mind, and that's where the next mental event will occur.

After you have grown familiar with observing mental images and thoughts—first by intentionally creating them and then by letting them arise of their own accord—continue observing the space of your mind and anything that arises within it. This mental space is not located in any specific physical region, and it doesn't have a center, a periphery, a size, or borders. When you begin to observe thoughts and images, you may find that they disappear as soon as you notice them. Be patient and relax more deeply. Then you will begin to discover a place of stillness within the motion of your mind. When we begin this practice, the normally agitated mind is like a snow globe that has just been shaken, and a flurry of memories and fantasies swirl around, swiftly emerging and disappearing. Settling the mind in its natural state involves letting all these mental activities arise without inhibiting, controlling, or modifying them in any way.

Throughout the course of daily life, many kinds of thoughts, emotions, and desires arise, and when our attention is focused outward to the world around us, our sensory experiences often obscure our inner life, just as the sun outshines the stars during the daytime. Those mental activities continue subconsciously even when we're not attending to them, and they exert a powerful influence on our lives. In this practice we open the Pandora's box of our minds and focus our full attention on whatever emerges from that inner space. Time and again when thoughts arise, you will immediately be swept up by them, and your attention will be carried away to the referents of those thoughts. For example, if a memory of a personal encounter from this morning arises, your attention will be focused on the people and circumstances involved. That's called daydreaming. In this practice, observe the thoughts and images of that memory as events in their own right—occurring here and now in the space of your mind—without letting your attention be carried back into the past. Likewise, when fantasies, worries, or expectations about the future arise, simply be aware of them in the present moment.

The mind is constantly in motion, but in the midst of the movements of thoughts and images there is a still space of awareness in which you can rest in the present moment, without being jerked around through space and time by the contents of your mind. This is the union of stillness and motion. Whatever events arise in your mind—be they pleasant or unpleasant, gentle or harsh, good or bad, long or short—just let them be. Observe them without distraction and without mentally grasping at them, pushing them away, identifying with them, or preferring for them to continue or disappear. Let your awareness be as neutral as space and as bright as a well-polished mirror. You are observing the face of your own mind, with all its blemishes, scars, and beauty marks. This is a direct path to self-knowledge.

At times you may begin to feel spaced out and unfocused. When that happens, revive your awareness by refocusing on the practice, training your attention clearly on the space of your mind and its contents. You may be peripherally aware of your breathing, and if so, let the in-breath be an occasion for focusing more intently on your mind. At other moments, you may find that you have been distracted and carried away by the contents of your mind. It's as if the space of your awareness had collapsed to the size of your thoughts and memories. As soon as you note that you are distracted, loosen up your body and mind and release your grasp on the thoughts that have captured your attention. This doesn't mean expelling the thoughts themselves. On the contrary, let them continue of their own accord for as long as they persist. But release the effort of identifying with them. It's especially easy to do this during the exhalation, a natural occasion for relaxing.

The kind of awareness we are bringing to the mind is discerning and intelligent, but also nonjudgmental. We are not evaluating one thought as being better or worse than another. You may find at times that you are compulsively engaging in a kind of internal commentary, as if you were the director trying to control what's happening, or at least a critic judging the performances of each of the actors. Give it a rest, and simply observe what's happening on the stage of your mind without commentary. And if internal judgments arise anyway, simply observe them; they too are contents of the mind and therefore grist for the mill.

As you continue settling the mind in its natural state, gradually the quantity of thoughts and images will subside. On occasion, you may not notice any contents at all. When that happens, closely observe the background of the empty space in which thoughts and images appear. Note whether it is a sheer nothingness or has any characteristics of its own. As you do so, you may begin to detect very subtle mental events that had previously escaped your notice. Because they are so subtle, they slip under the radar of ordinary consciousness. But now as the vividness and acuity of your attention are heightened, you may become aware of mental processes that had previously been locked within your subconscious. Some may persist for seconds at a time, barely crossing the threshold of consciousness because of their subtlety; others may flit across the space of your mind for only a fraction of a second. As your mindfulness become more and more continuous, you may detect these microevents for the first time.

You have now set out on one of the greatest expeditions as you explore the hidden recesses of your mind. Long-forgotten memories will emerge out of the blue, strange fantasies may haunt you, and the most bizarre thoughts and desires may lurch up and take you by surprise. Whatever thoughts and images arise, simply be aware of them, recognizing that they are only appearances to the mind. Observe them without being sucked into them. Passively but vigilantly let them arise from the space of your mind, and let them dissolve back into that space. Like reflections in a mirror, these thoughts and images have no power of their own to harm you or to help you. They are as insubstantial as mirages and rainbows, yet they have their own reality, as they causally interact among themselves and with your body. As you discover the luminous, still space of awareness in which the movements of the mind occur, you will begin to discover an inner freedom and place of rest even when the storms of turbulent emotions and desires sweep through this inner domain.

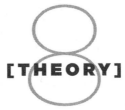

[THEORY]

KNOWING AND HEALING THE MIND

THE ORIGINS OF EVIL AND SUFFERING

According to the biblical account, suffering began with the original sin of Adam and Eve, and all subsequent generations of the human race have been blemished as if by a defective spiritual gene. The presence of evil in the world can therefore not be traced back to God, for even though he opened up the possibility of its occurrence by granting his creatures free will, he is not responsible for what we have freely chosen to do. The Bible states that God selected the people of Israel to be in a special relationship with him, but he still allowed them to suffer from various natural calamities such as famine, drought, and pestilence. For millennia theologians have struggled to understand this. Some have proposed that God was angry at his sinful, disobedient people and inflicted suffering on them for its redemptive value, to arouse humility, overcome pride, and test their faith. Others have suggested that God's ways are too mysterious for mere mortals to comprehend, but this implies that God can maim, torment, and murder at will and not be held accountable.

Within the Christian tradition, Saint Paul declared that God gave human beings over to our depraved minds, and of our own free will we have chosen to "become filled with every kind of wickedness, evil, greed, and depravity."[1] In terms of our innate human nature,

Paul insisted that none of us is righteous, but if we have faith in Jesus Christ, God's goodness may flow into and through us. God then rewards or punishes each person, Jew and Gentile alike, according to what we have done. To those who devote themselves to virtue, he grants eternal life, but those who are self-seeking and who reject the truth and follow evil will know God's wrath and anger.[2]

The Greek philosopher Epicurus (341–270 B.C.E.) was one of the earliest Western thinkers to reject belief in the immortality of the soul and divine reward and punishment in the hereafter. He refuted theistic answers regarding the origins of evil and suffering in the world with the argument: Is God willing to prevent evil but not able? Then he is impotent. Is he able but not willing? Then he is malevolent. Is he both able and willing? Whence, then, evil? In his view, all events in the world were ultimately based on the motions and interactions of atoms moving in empty space.

A very similar view had been proposed four centuries earlier by the Indian philosopher Charvaka. Like Epicurus, he believed that everything consists of the basic physical elements of nature. So human beings are simply physical organisms, and the mind is an emergent property of specific configurations of those elements that vanish at death. Charvaka taught that the ideal life holds pleasure as its goal, and this is to be gained by the accumulation of wealth and the pursuit of sensual and intellectual enjoyments. Ethics is simply what people subjectively decide upon, for there is nothing that is objectively right or wrong.[3]

Such beliefs have been widely embraced by atheists ever since. Freud, for example, pointed to three sources of suffering: "the superior power of nature, the feebleness of our own bodies and the inadequacy of the regulations which adjust the mutual relationships of human beings in the family, the state and society."[4] To battle the suffering caused by natural disasters and disease, he counseled, we must rely upon science, "going over to the attack against nature and subjecting her to the human will."[5] But because of our "own psychical constitution," we have a very limited capacity for virtue or happiness, so we must be satisfied with only a moderate degree of mental balance and well-being.[6]

A key element of the biblical account of the origins of evil and suffering is our God-given freedom of will, for without this, God appears to be a malevolent being who created the human race only to suffer, without taking any responsibility for his own role in our misery. Many contemporary biologists insist not only that God does not exist but also that free will is an illusion, for all human actions are caused solely by neurobiological events operating according to the laws of physics and chemistry.[7] This is a current version of the atomism of Epicurus. But there is no consensus on this point, for other neuroscientists have shown that studies of the brain and volition have not provided sufficient evidence to prove or disprove the existence of free will.[8]

Neuroscientists have clearly identified regions of the brain most closely correlated with emotions. The amygdala, which is a part of the limbic system located in the middle of the brain, is strongly associated with fear, anger, sadness, and disgust. But other emotions such as guilt and embarrassment are linked to neural activity in other parts of the brain, and the frontal cortex, which is closely related to reasoning abilities, is also closely related to emotions. When that area is damaged, one's ability to experience emotions of any kind may be seriously impaired. On the basis of such neuroscientific insights, the pharmaceutical industry has made great progress in developing a wide array of drugs designed to deactivate the neurobiological processes that regulate physical pain and mental suffering. Most of these drugs do nothing to eradicate the underlying cause of suffering, so in many cases they lead to long-term dependence, which may be a mixed blessing or even a curse. And this dependence can easily distract us from seeking out and addressing the primary causes of suffering.

One of the most widespread kinds of mental suffering today is depression, and despite the many drugs that have been created to treat its symptoms, an estimated 4 million Americans have depression that is resistant to chemical interventions. Even when antidepressant medications are effective, it has been shown that 50 to 75 percent of their efficacy is due to the placebo effect, or simple faith in the effectiveness of the treatment. Such faith brings about changes in the brain different from those associated with antidepressant medication, but these changes still alleviate the misery of depression.[9] The power of faith, or belief, has also been proven to alleviate physical suffering while producing physical changes in areas of the brain associated with such discomfort. While the power of faith, known as the placebo effect, can produce health benefits, the "nocebo effect" can lead to the opposite. When people expect they will experience something painful or afflictive, that's just what happens. In this case as well, their thoughts, emotions, and beliefs cause physical effects in the brain, but the nature of these mind-body causal interactions is far from clear.

What is evident is that the human mind plays a dominant role in the origins of evil and suffering. Saint Augustine declared that the two primary causes of misery are "the love of things vain and noxious" and "the profundity of ignorance."[10] The Buddhist tradition also identifies craving and ignorance as the root causes of evil and suffering, and though Christian and Buddhist contemplatives certainly have different ideas about the exact nature of those causes, in principle their diagnoses of the source of misery converge on the workings of the human mind. Regarding the origins of good and evil, joy and sorrow, the Buddha declared, "All things are preceded by the mind, issue forth from the mind, and consist of the mind."[11] Given the primacy of the mind's role in the pursuit of genuine happiness and meaning, it deserves the most careful observation, which can be done with sustained contemplative practice.

OBSERVING THE MIND

Within the biblical context, the practice of quietly observing the mind may be understood in relation to the third commandment: "Remember the Sabbath day, to keep it holy." Augustine declared that this commandment encourages us to cultivate a quietness of the heart and a tranquility of the mind. "This is holiness," he wrote, "because here is the Spirit of God. This is what a true holiday means, quietness and rest . . . we are offered a kind of Sabbath in the heart." He continued that it is as if God were saying, "'Stop being so restless, quiet the uproar in your minds. Let go of the idle fantasies that fly around in your head.' God is saying, 'Be still and see that I am God' (Psalms 46)."[12]

This meditative practice was clearly taught by Evagrius of Pontus, who offered guidance to the aspiring contemplative: "Let him keep careful watch over his thoughts. Let him observe their intensity, their periods of decline and follow them as they rise and fall. Let him note well the complexity of his thoughts, their periodicity, the demons which cause them, with the order of their succession and the nature of their associations."[13] Regarding the dispassionate awareness of thoughts and feelings, Evagrius taught his students to quietly observe thoughts and feelings without becoming immersed in them.[14] Greek Orthodox contemplatives preserved this tradition of building self-awareness by observing the mind, in which we cultivate qualities of watchfulness (*nepsis*) and discernment (*diakrisis*), which enable us to distinguish between good and evil thoughts.[15] As the contemporary scholar Martin Laird eloquently writes, such practice continues to this day among Christian contemplatives: "It can be rather painful as repressed material comes into awareness, what Thomas Keating has called 'the unloading of the unconscious.'[16] But this is the essence of liberating integration: allowing into awareness what was previously kept out of awareness. Until we can see this, we will not see that there is something utterly vast and sacred already within us, this silent land that runs deeper than these obsessive mental patterns."[17]

Buddhism too has a long and highly developed tradition of observing the mind. One method the Buddha taught for counteracting distraction was to focus the attention on some worthy object, and then to release that object and simply be inwardly mindful and at ease, without actively engaging in any thinking or active inquiry.[18] A skillful practitioner, he said, concentrates and purifies the mind by clearly apprehending its characteristics, but without such discerning awareness, the mind is neither concentrated nor purified.[19]

The practice of settling the mind in its natural state has been especially emphasized in the Mahayana tradition, as it gradually spread from India to Nepal and on to Tibet. The eleventh-century Nepalese Buddhist contemplative Maitripa, for instance, taught the practice of steadily observing whatever virtuous and nonvirtuous thoughts arise in the mind, without desire or aversion. In this way, he declared, thoughts subside of their own accord, and clear, empty awareness vividly arises without any object other than itself.[20] Panchen Lozang Chökyi Gyaltsen (1570–1662), the tutor of the Fifth Dalai Lama of Tibet, explained this practice as follows:

> Whatever sorts of thoughts arise, without suppressing them, recognize what they emerge from and what they dissolve into; and stay focused while you observe their nature. By doing so, eventually the motion of thoughts ceases and there is stillness . . . each time you observe the nature of any thoughts that arise, they will vanish by themselves, following which, a vacuity appears. Likewise, if you also examine the mind when it remains without movement, you will see an unobscured, clear and vivid vacuity, without any difference between the former and latter states. That is well known among meditators and is called "the union of stillness and motion."[21]

This practice has long been embraced by the Great Perfection (Dzogchen) school of Tibetan Buddhism, which is focused on fathoming the nature of awareness. Düdjom Lingpa (1835–1904), one of the greatest nineteenth-century contemplatives in the tradition, wrote that this kind of meditation is especially suitable for people with stressed-out bodies and agitated, coarse minds.[22] That seems to characterize virtually everyone in the modern world! "Such people," he wrote, "should relax and let thoughts be as they are, continually observing them with unwavering mindfulness and careful introspection."[23] In this way, the movements of thoughts do not cease, but when one doesn't get lost in them as usual, they are illuminated by mindful awareness. He continued, "By applying yourself to this practice constantly at all times, both during and between meditation sessions, eventually all coarse and subtle thoughts will be calmed in the empty expanse of the essential nature of your mind. You will become still in an unfluctuating state, in which you will experience joy like the warmth of a fire, clarity like the dawn, and nonconceptuality like an ocean unmoved by waves."[24] His description of this practice is so lucid that it deserves to be cited at length:

Appearances and awareness become simultaneous, so events seem to be released as soon as they are witnessed. Thus, emergence and release are simultaneous. As soon as things emerge from their own space, they are released back into their own space, like lightning flashing from the sky and vanishing back into the sky. Since this appears by looking within, it is called liberation in the expanse. All these are in fact the unification and single-pointed focus of mindfulness and appearances. After all pleasant and unpleasant experiential visions have dissolved into absolute space, consciousness rests in its own stainless, radiant clarity. Whatever thoughts and memories arise, do not cling to these experiences; do not modify or judge them, but let them arise as they rove to and fro. In doing so, the effort of vivid, steady apprehension—as in the case of thoughts apprehended by tight mindfulness—vanishes of its own accord. Such effort makes the unsatiated mind compulsively strive after mental objects. Sometimes, feeling dissatisfied as if you're lacking something, you may compulsively engage in a lot of mental activity entailing tight concentration and so on. In this phase, consciousness comes to rest in its own state, mindfulness emerges, and because there is less clinging to experiences, consciousness settles into its own natural, unmodified state. In this way you come to a state of naturally settled mindfulness. That experience is soothing and gentle, with clear, limpid consciousness that is neither benefited nor harmed by thoughts; and you experience a remarkable sense of stillness without needing to modify, reject, or embrace anything.[25]

Although the Christian and Buddhist accounts of this practice have much in common, there seem to be significant differences in their underlying assumptions and their interpretations of the benefits of such meditation. Augustine expressed the view of many Christians in his assertion that the soul cannot be happy through a goodness of its own, because it must look "outside itself" for perfection, which can be found only in the changeless, which is God.[26] Later contemplatives in the Roman Catholic and Greek Orthodox traditions likewise emphasized that the benefits of meditation are not due to one's own efforts but depend entirely on grace.[27] The self is depicted as a wretched sinner whose corrupt nature requires outside, divine intervention in order to be saved.

The Buddhist tradition, in contrast, has always declared that the mind is not intrinsically defiled or afflicted and that liberation may be achieved through one's own efforts. This point was clearly made by the Buddha himself just before he passed into nirvana, when he told his disciples, "live as islands unto yourselves, being your own refuge with no one else as your refuge."[28] As much as the mind may be habitually polluted by afflictive thoughts and emotions, its essential nature is pure and luminous, so the mind is capable of healing itself without any outside intervention by a higher power.

On the surface, this appears to be a fundamental difference between Christianity and Buddhism, but let's probe a bit more deeply. When raising the question of whether we must seek outside ourselves for happiness and liberation, it is important to ask, what are the boundaries of the self? Insofar as I identify myself with my body, it has the skin to separate it from the outside. I may also identify myself with my mental activities, including thoughts, mental images, emotions, intentions, desires, memories, fantasies, and dreams. Clearly, the benefits of settling the mind into its natural state do not result from "my" doing anything to the mind. Rather, I am simply observing events arising and passing in the mind, without trying to alter any of them. So the benefits of this practice are not created by myself as the thinker, but instead occur spontaneously as the mind gradually settles in its own calm, luminous, ground state. If I regard that space of inner purity to be outside myself, or to belong to God, then the benefits from this practice can be attributed to grace. But if I view that space as a deeper dimension of my own being, then I don't need to look outside myself for liberation. So who draws the boundaries between what is inside and outside the self? I believe that we do, just as we define all the rest of the words in our vocabulary and thereby mark the boundaries of the referents of those words.

Descartes is best known for his assertion, "I think, therefore I am," implying an "egocentric" view of thoughts and other mental activities.[29] In this practice, however, we challenge the assumption that we are the agents responsible for the generation of every thought, image, desire, and emotion that arises in our minds. Anyone who ventures into this method for observing the mind quickly discovers that many mental processes arise of their own accord, without any active participation by oneself as the agent. You are simply a disengaged observer, passively witnessing events arise and pass within the space of your mind, recognizing that many thoughts arise without a thinker.[30] Such mental events are viewed as natural phenomena that emerge from moment to moment in dependence upon prior physical and psychological causes. Further, by carefully observing our minds in this way, we get out of the rut of compulsively assuming that our thoughts and mental images of people and events accurately and completely represent them as they exist independently of our own perspective and experience. This is truly liberating.

All the great revolutions in the physical and life sciences have been based on the direct, meticulous observation of the phenomena under investigation. The practice of settling the mind in its natural state allows for the dispassionate, "objective" observation of mental phenomena, including the whole array of subjectively experienced mental states and events. To qualify as a rigorous method of scientific inquiry, this observation must be free of subjective biases related to personal assumptions, emotions, desires, and fears, just like any other kind of scientific observation. Moreover, this practice is objective in the sense that the ego is largely removed from the picture as we do our best to set aside our preconceptions and biases.

Settling the mind in its natural state is not only an effective way of knowing the mind but also has great potential for healing the mind. We already know that the body has a remarkable capacity to heal. Whether it is injured by an abrasion or a bone fracture or being assailed by harmful bacteria and viruses, the body has an astonishing ability to mend its wounds and cleanse itself of injurious agents from the environment. But for this to happen, it often needs help, as in keeping a wound clean and bandaged, setting a broken bone, or surgically removing contaminated tissue. The body and mind are so intimately connected that it's reasonable to hypothesize that the mind too has a great capacity to heal itself. The problem is that when the mind is wounded—by trauma from a natural disaster, social conflict, or illness, by other people's abuse, or even by our own harmful behavior—we often let those wounds fester. The mind obsessively churns up memories of the past or speculations about the future and we compulsively fixate and elaborate on them in ways that aggravate our mental afflictions. Psychologists call this tendency rumination, and it's a way that mental wounds become infected, which obstructs the natural healing capacity of the mind.

In this practice you "surgically remove" the mental habits of 1) thinking that the thoughts and images you experience exist outside of your own mind, 2) compulsively responding to those mental events with craving and aversion, as if they were intrinsically pleasant or unpleasant in and of themselves, and 3) identifying with them as if you are the independent agent who created them, while viewing them as intrinsically "yours" simply because you alone experience them. Scientists excel at understanding natural phenomena that can be examined repeatedly by multiple observers. But phenomena that are unique to a particular time (and therefore not repeatable) and to a particular individual (such as your thoughts) are no less real. Moreover, the mere fact that something is observed by yourself alone doesn't necessarily make it yours. For example, if you enjoy a beautiful sunset all by yourself, you can't lay claim to it as your possession. You were simply in the right place at the right time to witness it. The same is true of all subjective experience. It can't be directly observed by anyone else, but that doesn't make it any less real than public events, nor does it imply that we are personally responsible for everything we witness as we observe the space of our minds.

This transition from an egocentric to a naturalistic view of mental phenomena can be wonderfully liberating. For in this process of carefully observing mental events without distraction and without grasping, we begin to see how the mind can heal itself. We are keeping the wounds of the mind clean, and—whether we attribute this to grace from a supernatural being or to the natural quality of awareness—many of the knots of the mind begin to untangle by themselves. This practice is not suggested as a cure-all or as a substitute for professionally administered therapy. At times, such outside intervention is necessary. But there appears to be great potential for combining this practice with such intervention in ways that will enable people with psychological problems to enter more fully into a partnership with their therapist to restore and enhance their mental health. Such "cross-cultural" therapy is a new and rapidly growing field of clinical research that bears great promise for the future.[31]

MINDFULNESS AND INTROSPECTION

The purpose of the practice of settling the mind in its natural state is to cultivate a deepening sense of physical and mental ease, stillness, and vigilance. This is achieved by using and refining the two mental faculties of mindfulness and introspection. As mentioned in an earlier chapter, psychologists have recently been studying the effects of mindfulness, defined as "a kind of nonelaborative, nonjudgmental, present-centered awareness in which each thought, feeling, or sensation that arises in the attentional field is acknowledged and accepted as it is."[32] That's a good description of the kind of awareness we bring to this practice, although not really equivalent to the meaning of mindfulness as it is presented in the Buddhist tradition. In the Pali language, in which the Buddha's teachings were first recorded, the term we translate as "mindfulness" is *sati*, which the Buddha defined as the ability "to remember, to keep in memory what was said and done long ago."[33] So the primary Buddhist meaning of mindfulness is recollection, which is the opposite of forgetfulness. When we apply mindfulness to observing the mind, we "recollect" our attention from moment to moment as we observe the ongoing flow of events that arise and pass, without succumbing to forgetfulness.

Possibly the earliest attempt in Buddhist literature to fully explain the meaning of *sati* is found in a dialogue between Menander I (second century B.C.E.), an Indo-Greek king of northwestern India, and Nagasena, a Buddhist sage who had received his own training from the Greek Buddhist monk Dhammarakkhita. When questioned by the king about the nature of mindfulness, Nagasena replied that it has both the characteristic of "calling to mind" and the characteristic of "taking hold." He explained further, "Mindfulness, when it arises, calls to mind wholesome and unwholesome tendencies, with faults and faultless, inferior and refined, dark and pure, together with their counterparts. . . . Mindfulness, when it arises, follows the courses of beneficial and unbeneficial tendencies: these tendencies are beneficial, these unbeneficial; these tendencies are helpful, these unhelpful."[34]

This theme was picked up again by the fifth-century Indian Buddhist scholar Buddhaghosa, the most authoritative commentator in the Theravada tradition of Buddhism, which is preserved nowadays primarily in Southeast Asia. In his classic work, *The Path of Purification,* he begins his explanation of this topic by commenting that it is by means of mindfulness that we are able to recall things or events in the past. It has the characteristic, he writes, of "not floating," in that the mind is closely engaged with the chosen object of attention. It has the property of "not losing," indicating that mindfulness enables us to maintain our attention without forgetfulness. It manifests in "guarding" or being "face to face with the object," implying that "the rope of mindfulness" holds the attention firmly to its chosen object, whether it is a relatively stable single object or a continuum of events. Its basis is "strong noting," suggesting its discerning quality. In summary, he comments that mindfulness should be seen as like a post due to its state of being set in the object, and as like a gatekeeper because it guards the doors of perception.[35]

While engaging in the practice of settling the mind in its natural state, we do not try to alter any of its contents but simply observe whatever arises with unwavering mindfulness. But in the course of our daily lives, mindfulness can play a more active role, as suggested by Nagasena and Buddhaghosa, in helping to cultivate wholesome mental states and alleviate unwholesome ones. Just as a gatekeeper prevents those not entitled from entering a town, so does well-established mindfulness prevent the arising of unwholesome associations and reactions to the physical senses. Many Buddhist treatises describe mindfulness as the one factor that guards the mind,[36] or as a mental faculty that exerts a controlling influence on thoughts and intentions.[37] So it is incorrect to assume that mindfulness is always passive.

In the Buddhist context of meditation, mindfulness has the connotation of contemplation, in the sense of "to see" or "to closely observe." Clearly, this is a very close match to the Latin *contemplatio* and the Greek *theoria,* which also mean "to contemplate" and "to observe." Like the Pythagoreans and the Christian contemplative tradition, the Buddha emphasized the importance of mindfulness for all types of meditation, because mindfulness forms the essential condition for "contemplation" and "knowledge."[38]

When one is settling the mind in its natural state, the object of mindfulness is the space of the mind and whatever mental activities arise there. In order for this practice to be effective, however, we also need to apply and refine another mental faculty, introspection. In the Buddhist tradition, introspection is defined as the repeated examination of the state of one's body and mind, and it is regarded as a kind of discerning intelligence.[39] The Buddhist understanding of mindfulness and introspection therefore bears a strong resemblance to the Christian understanding of watchfulness and discernment.

The two major attentional imbalances we tend to encounter when engaging in meditative practice are laxity and excitation. When laxity sets in, the mind loses its clarity and we become spaced out or simply fall into a dull, sluggish state on the way to falling asleep. When excitation arises, the mind becomes distracted and agitated, making it difficult to sustain our attention on anything with continuity. Both laxity and excitation result in a loss of mindfulness, by the attention either collapsing in on itself or being compulsively propelled outward. With the faculty of introspection we monitor the quality of our attention, noting as swiftly as possible when either of these imbalances occurs. Buddhaghosa clarified the relationship between the two: "Mindfulness has the characteristic of remembering. Its function is not to forget. It is manifested as guarding. Introspection has the characteristic of non-confusion. Its function is to investigate. It is manifested as scrutiny."[40] In other words, with mindfulness we focus continually, without forgetfulness, on the mind, and with introspection we closely examine whether the attention has been caught up in laxity or excitation. Thus, introspection "looks over mindfulness' shoulder."

Simply recognizing that our attention is getting dull or agitated is not enough. As soon as we notice this, we need to exert the right amount of effort to overcome the imbalance. This is an act of will. When we recognize that laxity has arisen, the immediate remedy is to take a fresh interest in the object of mindfulness. In this case, we apply more effort as we sharpen the focus of attention. In the other case, as soon as we note that the mind has become distracted and is caught up in thoughts, the antidote is to relax a bit, both physically and mentally. No matter what comes up, we simply attend to it with unwavering mindfulness.

To support this practice, in between sessions it is useful to apply mindfulness and introspection to more actively transform the mind by cultivating wholesome mental states and rejecting thoughts and other impulses that are harmful to ourselves and others. This is what Nagasena was getting at when he said that mindfulness follows the courses of wholesome and unwholesome mental tendencies, recognizing their beneficial and harmful effects. This is also what Buddhaghosa meant when he referred to mindfulness as being like a gatekeeper that guards the doors of perception. The mind can be one of the most destructive forces in nature, and when we recognize that it's running amok, it's only sensible to restrain it, and we do this with mindfulness.

In terms of offering guidance for a lifestyle that supports meditative practice, traditional Buddhist sources cite four elements: ethical discipline, restraint of the sense faculties, mindfulness and introspection, and contentment.[41] Basic requisites for such training also include a suitable diet, clothing, and, when needed, medication. Ethical discipline consists of doing our best to avoid behavior that is injurious to ourselves and others. When our physical senses roam to objects that upset the equilibrium of the mind by arousing craving or hostility, it can be helpful to restrain our senses and focus our attention directly on our own mental processes so as to understand them better. This doesn't overcome the tendencies toward craving and hostility, but at least it helps keep us from digging deeper into these ruts. Mindfulness and introspection are useful at all times, not just during meditation, for remaining engaged with reality instead of being caught up in our fantasies and slipping into dull-mindedness. And contentment with the basic necessities of life is the key to pursuing genuine happiness, which comes from within, rather than from pleasant stimuli. With these basic components, our meditative practice and our daily lives gradually merge, and the distinction between formal meditation and ordinary activities throughout the day begins to fade. Even in the midst of an active way of life we may discover an inner silence, and this deepens our sense of the union of stillness and motion.

REFLECTIONS OF THE MIND

As we venture into the practice of settling the mind in its natural state, we may wonder: what is the nature of these appearances that arise in the space of the mind, and what do they tell us about the nature of the mind itself? The best way to gain insight into these appearances is to observe them carefully. Astronomers have learned about the stars and planets by careful observation, and biologists have learned about plants and animals the same way. Thoughts, mental images, desires, and emotions arise from the hidden recesses of the mind, influenced by physiological processes in our bodies and experiences in this lifetime and possibly past lifetimes. When we identify with them, they have a powerful influence on our bodies, minds, and behavior. However, when we simply observe them, as taught in the last practice, we can learn from them without falling under their domination. These appearances can tell us about our unconscious hopes and fears, and they reveal the creative potentials of the luminous space of the mind from which they arise.

Although many people believe that subjective experience must be equivalent to brain activity, this has never been demonstrated scientifically, and there are good reasons to doubt this assumption. Imagine, for example, that you have just spoken gently to someone who was very upset, and you were able to calm this person by speaking with sensitivity and kindness. Afterward you may feel glad that you were able to help them. When that experience of gladness arises, specific configurations of neural activity are certainly taking place in your brain. But if that brain activity were artificially induced with drugs, for instance, it wouldn't correspond to the same mental state. For the emotion you felt after helping someone would be more *meaningful* than a similar emotion generated chemically. Brain activity provides only a partial explanation for the kinds of subjective experiences we have from moment to moment, and any attempt to reduce mental processes to brain activity always leaves out something crucial: the *mental* processes themselves!

Descartes maintained that the primary quality of physical entities is that they are extended in space, that is, they have definite locations and spatial dimensions. Many people think that thoughts are actually inside our heads, because that's where their neural correlates are located. But we know that physical effects sometimes occur far from their causes, and physical causation does not always require tangible objects to bump into each other. Descartes, with his mechanistic view of the universe, believed that such physical contact was always necessary (except when the mind interacts with the body), but modern physics has abandoned this assumption. For example, when two electromagnetic fields traveling through space interact with each other, creating interference patterns, the collision cannot be understood in mechanical terms. And in quantum mechanics, many physical interactions occur at a distance, with no collisions of particles acting like tiny billiard balls.

If we take modern physics into account and move beyond Descartes' outdated view of reality, we are not compelled to believe that mental events are actually located inside the brain simply because that's where their neural correlates are.[42] Moreover, it doesn't necessarily follow that something has to be physical simply because it is influenced by physical processes and exerts its own effects on other physical entities. Although this is still widely believed by people who are unfamiliar with contemporary physics, it is no longer accepted by scientists as a hard and fast law governing the whole of nature.

If mental processes are physical, they should have physical qualities, such as location, spatial dimensions, and mass, and it should be possible to detect them with at least some of the many instruments of technology designed to measure all known kinds of physical entities. But however closely scientists examine the brain, they never see any mental events, just interactions of chemicals and electricity. And however closely contemplatives observe their own minds, they don't seem to detect any brain mechanisms that cause the mental processes they are experiencing. In fact, the more closely we investigate brain and mental processes, the clearer it becomes that they have very little in common except that they are interrelated. This is presumably why Christof Koch, as mentioned above, has expressed skepticism that mental processes can ever be understood as nothing more than activities in the brain.[43]

The question remains, though: can we really know the nature of the mind by examining the appearances of thoughts and other mental processes? After all, many sensory appearances are illusory. The Earth, for instance, appears to be flat; the Sun appears to circle around the Earth; and there are many other optical illusions in nature, such as mirages. Why should we credit our own direct experience of our minds when they may be fundamentally misleading? This same qualm could be raised, however, with regard to *all* our direct experience. As Descartes rightly pointed out, colors, sounds, smells, tastes, and tactile sensations all seem to exist in the objective world, independently of our experience of them. But these appearances are illusory. Photons and electromagnetic fields, which are the objective basis for our experience of colors, don't have any colors of their own. Colors arise only in dependence upon a conscious subject perceiving those photons and electromagnetic fields. Likewise, sounds don't exist objectively in the ripples in a medium such as air or water, and smells and tastes don't exist in the air or in food independently of someone experiencing them. But if scientists refused to examine these appearances simply because they are illusory, they would never learn anything about the world around us! Galileo would not have given any credit to the visual appearances that were the bases of his many discoveries about the Sun, Moon, planets, and stars, and Darwin wouldn't have taken seriously his many biological observations that provided that the basis for his theory of evolution.

The whole history of science demonstrates that we learn about the world by carefully observing appearances and then reasoning out our observations. When we attend to mental phenomena as we settle the mind in its natural state, we are following in the footsteps of generations of scientists who have explored the external world by carefully observing what appeared to their physical senses. But here's one big difference: Galileo was able to extend his visual perception with the telescope, and later generations of scientists and engineers have devised many technological means of extending our physical senses to explore the world outside us in greater detail. But none of those instruments can detect a single mental process. The only way that mental activities can be detected is by observing the mind with mental awareness. And when we do so, it's apparent that mental states and processes don't bear any of the qualities that Descartes uniquely attribute to physical entities. So we have two good reasons for assuming that mental events aren't physical: they can't be detected with any of the instruments of technology, which are designed to measure all known kinds of physical entities, and when we do observe mental phenomena, they don't appear to have any physical characteristics.

As we progress in settling the mind in its natural state, it becomes more and more obvious that the mind is not one unified thing. At first, thoughts may vanish as soon as we observe them, or we may notice them only after we have been carried away by them. But as we become more experienced in this technique, we start to notice that some mental events, like discursive thoughts and mental images, have a kind of objective quality. We have a sense of observing them "over there" in the space of our minds. The same is true of objects we perceive in a dream. If I dream of being in a room full of people, the room and the people appear as objects of my awareness, as do the internal chitchat and mental images that arise in meditation.

We may also detect emotions and desires that have a more subjective quality: they don't appear so much as objects to our mental awareness, but as qualities of that awareness. By quietly being aware of but not totally absorbed by them, we can remain aware of the larger context in which those emotions and desires arose. In other words, we can see the forest as a whole and not confine our awareness to individual trees. When our very identity fuses with such a restrictive mental impulse, we can literally become "small-minded," and that can lead to a lot of regrettable behavior. We observe mental images at the same time as they arise in the mind, but when we experience emotions and desires, we may actually be recollecting a mental state that just slipped by. For example, when you feel resentful that someone has treated you thoughtlessly, your attention is focused on that person's behavior. But as soon you direct your attention to that resentment, it's no longer being fed by thinking about the offensive person, so it may immediately fade away. When an emotion or a desire arises, the mind is usually focused on the object of those mental states, rather than the emotion or desire itself. This is probably what William James had in mind when he wrote, "No subjective state, whilst present, is its own object; its object is always something else. . . . The act of naming them has momentarily detracted from their force."[44] This raises fascinating questions about the impact of observing the mind. For example, if you are depressed, does your depression diminish by your act of observing it? This you should check out for yourself. Sometimes, especially if the depression is a passing emotion about something that happened recently, you may find that it vanishes as soon as you pay close attention to it. But if you have settled into a lingering mood of depression, with no particular object in mind, you may find that it persists even while you attend to it. Still, you may not feel so trapped if you are objectively aware of it and recognize it as a state of mind, not an intrinsic quality of yourself. Likewise, if you observe the presence of a desire arising in your mind, does it immediately lose its force as a result of your awareness of it? If it's a powerful, habitual desire, it may remain even while you focus on it. But if it's a fleeting desire that arose because of a specific thought or sensory experience, it may disappear. The effect of your awareness on your thoughts, emotions, and desires is worth spending a lot of time investigating. The practice of settling the mind can be wonderfully liberating as you recognize more and more clearly that you are not identical to these mental activities.

Descartes commented that when he observed the appearances to his own mind, he perceived them with such obscurity and confusion that he did not even know whether they were true. This is certainly the experience of many people when they begin settling the mind in its natural state. But a remarkable quality of mental awareness is that it can be refined with training. At the beginning of this practice, we may perceive only the most superficial and coarse mental events, but as we delve deeper and deeper into it—especially when we practice for many hours a day for days or weeks in succession—we may perceive increasingly subtle and brief events distinctly and clearly. In this process of refining mental awareness, we are bringing previously subconscious elements of the mind—such as old memories, emotions, and desires—into the light of consciousness. The exploration of the hidden reaches of the mind has begun.

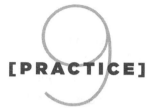

[PRACTICE]

BEHOLD THE LIGHT OF CONSCIOUSNESS

Settle your body in a comfortable position, sitting on a chair, sitting cross-legged, or lying down. Be still and vigilant, and take three slow, deep breaths, experiencing the sensations of the breath throughout your body. Then settle your respiration in its natural rhythm, letting your body determine whether your breathing is deep or shallow, slow or fast, regular or irregular. Now rest your mind in open, choiceless awareness, letting your attention roam to any of your six senses (the five physical senses and the mind) without trying to control it in any way. If a sound catches your attention, let your awareness rest on that, without fixating on it or withdrawing from it. Likewise, if some visual impression or bodily sensation arises to your awareness, simply be present with it, without getting caught up in or identifying with it. When you notice thoughts, memories, or other mental events, let your attention alight on them like a butterfly touching down on a flower, without clinging to them. For a few minutes, rest in this spacious sense of awareness in which you give up all sense of controlling your mind.

Now begin to withdraw your attention by focusing exclusively on the space of your body, noticing any kind of sensation that arises there, from the tips of your toes to the crown of your head. Instead of letting the wild steed of your mind roam at will through all the six sense fields (including the mental domain), corral it within the confines of your body. But within that space, continue to let your mind come to rest on any sensation that catches your attention. And simply be present with it, without getting caught up in or trying to control it in any way.

After a few minutes, withdraw your attention even further, into the space of your mind (as in the last practice) taking note of the mental events that arise and pass away there. Observe the contents of your mind, such as discursive thoughts and images, as they objectively arise to your awareness from moment to moment. Be aware too of impulses such as emotions and desires that you experience subjectively, and continue to rest in the open space of your awareness without identifying with them. Just be aware of them, not trying to modify or react to them.

By attending to these objective contents and subjective impulses, you have focused on the "foreground" of your mind. Now shift your attention to the "background," from which these mental events emerge, in which they play themselves out, and into which they finally dissolve. Carefully observe this mental space and note whether it has any characteristics of its own or is simply nothingness.

Now for the final step in this meditation: in all the previous exercises, you have focused your attention on some *thing*, either in one of your five physical sense fields or in your mind. Your attention has been like a laser pointer directed at the screens of your fields of experience, illuminating them. Now retract that laser pointer into itself. Withdraw your attention into its own nature without taking an interest in anything else, not even the space of the mind or its contents. Let your awareness rest in its own space, and simply be aware of being aware. Whatever objects appear to your consciousness, let them be, without trying to shut them out. Just don't take an interest in them. As soon as they tug your attention outward, release them and let your awareness rest in its own nature. Whenever a thought arises, release it immediately and let your mind settle in a nonconceptual mode of quiet, still awareness.

As simple as this practice sounds, at the beginning you may find it a bit difficult. If so, you may conjoin this practice with your breath. During each inhalation, draw your awareness in upon itself and simply experience the present moment of consciousness. With each out-breath, immediately release any thoughts or other distractions that may have caught your attention while continuing to be aware of the experience of being aware. With each in-breath, arouse your attention, overcoming laxity and dullness, and with each out-breath, relax your attention, overcoming excitation and agitation.

Your knowledge of being aware may be the most certain knowledge you have. It is the knowing of knowing, the awareness that awareness is happening, right here, right now. Maintain a close, vigilant awareness of awareness and see if you can discern its qualities. Is it still or flowing? Does it have spatial dimensions, large or small? Does it have a shape, a center, or boundaries? If it does have a size or shape, does that change or remain constant? Finally, can you identify unique characteristics of consciousness that belong to nothing else?

In this practice, you sustain mindfulness of awareness itself, but it is also important to exercise your faculty of introspection, monitoring the quality of your attention. With introspection you note whether your mind has fallen into laxity, and as soon as that happens, you may counteract it—arousing your attention by taking a renewed interest in awareness. When through introspection you notice that your mind has become caught up in distracting thoughts or other stimuli, immediately relax and let go of those objects of the mind. It takes effort to maintain your grip on those distractions, so release that effort as well as the objects that distract you, and let your awareness return home. This is like settling into a deep, dreamless sleep. But instead of gradually losing the clarity of awareness as you normally do when you fall asleep, you maintain a high level of vigilance. As you become more and more familiar with this practice, you may gradually unveil the stillness and luminosity that are intrinsic to awareness. Then you will no longer need to remedy agitation or dullness, for you will no longer be caught up in mental states that obscure the underlying nature of consciousness.

Continue for twenty-five minutes, then bring the session to a close. As you become more and more familiar with this practice, you may gradually increase the duration of your sessions, but don't let them last so long that the quality of your meditation decreases. It's helpful to have a meditation timer that lets you know when your session is over, so you don't need to interrupt your practice by glancing at a clock. For as long as you are meditating, do your best to maintain clear, unwavering mindfulness.

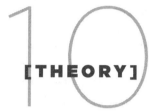

[THEORY]

EXPLORING THE NATURE OF CONSCIOUSNESS

CHRISTIAN EXPLORATIONS

Directing awareness inward to illuminate itself is a practice that has been used for centuries in various contemplative traditions in the East and the West. Within Christianity, it can be traced back to the Desert Fathers meditating in Egypt during the early centuries of the Christian church. Hesychios the Priest (seventh century), for example, a priest and monk who lived in a monastery on Mount Sinai, commented on this form of meditation in his treatise *On Watchfulness and Holiness*. A central theme of this meditation manual is attentiveness, which he defined as "the heart's stillness, unbroken by any thought."[1] "When the heart has acquired stillness," he wrote, "it will perceive the heights and depths of knowledge; and the ear of the still intellect will be made to hear marvelous things from God."[2] This gives rise to a unique kind of spiritual well-being.

The meditative practice of turning awareness upon itself was preserved by Greek Orthodox hermits from the tenth to the fourteenth centuries. The monk Saint Symeon (949–1022), for instance, counseled aspiring contemplatives to first of all seek three things: to free themselves of all anxiety regarding both real and imaginary things; to strive for a pure conscience, with no lingering sense of self-reproach; and to be completely detached, so that one's thoughts are not drawn to anything worldly, not even to one's own body.[3] Then, after withdrawing one's awareness from all worldly concerns, the attention is focused on one's heart and the practice continues as follows:

> To start with you will find there darkness and an impenetrable density. Later, when you persist and practice this task day and night, you will find, as though miraculously, an unceasing joy. For as soon as the intellect attains the place of the heart, at once it sees things of which it previously knew nothing. It sees the open space within the heart and it beholds itself entirely luminous and full of discrimination. From then on, from whatever side a distractive thought may appear, before it has come to completion and assumed a form, the intellect immediately drives it away and destroys it with the invocation of Jesus Christ. . . . The rest you will learn for yourself, with God's help, by keeping guard over your intellect and by retaining Jesus in your heart. As the saying goes, "Sit in your cell and it will teach you everything."[4]

Nikiphoros the Monk lived in the second half of the thirteenth century and dwelled in stillness on the Holy Mountain of Athos. In his treatise "On Watchfulness and the Guarding of the Heart," he emphasized the need to turn inward, letting one's awareness descend into the depths of the heart to discover the hidden treasure of the inner kingdom. Saint Gregory Palamas (1296–1359), who spent twenty years in monastic seclusion on the Holy Mountain, also encouraged those who sought "a life of self-attentiveness and stillness to bring their intellect back and to enclose it within their body, and particularly within that innermost body within the body that we call the heart."[5] But he made clear that all references to one's awareness descending into the heart are not to be interpreted literally, for our mental faculties, he wrote, are not located spatially inside the physical heart "as in a container."[6]

Although Christian contemplative inquiry into the nature of awareness has steadily declined with the rise of modernity, it has not vanished entirely. As late as the nineteenth century, the Russian Orthodox monk Saint Theophan the Recluse (1815–94) referred to this practice when he wrote, "Images, however sacred they may be, retain the attention outside, whereas at the time of prayer the attention must be within—in the heart. The concentration of attention in the heart—this is the starting point of prayer."[7] And the contemporary American contemplative scholar Martin Laird clearly describes it as follows:

Shift your awareness from the distraction to the awareness itself, to the aware-ing. There is nothing but this same luminous vastness, this depthless depth. What gazes into luminous vastness is itself luminous vastness. There is not a separate self who is afraid or angry or jealous. Clearly fear, anger, jealousy may be present, but we won't find anyone who is afraid, angry, jealous, etc., just luminous, depthless depth gazing into luminous, depthless depth.[8]

As a result of such practice, Christian contemplatives through the ages have reported exceptional states of inner knowledge and genuine well-being—a kind of "truth-given joy"—that arise when the heart is purified and brought to rest in its own innermost depths.

TWENTIETH-CENTURY INSIGHTS INTO CONSCIOUSNESS

From the early seventeenth century onward, while scientists confined their research to the external world, the inner world of the human soul and consciousness was left to theologians and philosophers. Despite their many ingenious theories, they failed to come to a consensus on even the most rudimentary questions, and in the late nineteenth century scientists began to investigate this unexplored dimension of the natural world. William James was fascinated by this topic, as it can be viewed from scientific, philosophical, and spiritual perspectives, and he rejected the notion that all physical and mental phenomena arise out of some primal stuff called "matter." In his view, the primal substance of the universe is pure experience, which he characterized as "plain, unqualified actuality, or existence, a simple *that*," prior to the differentiation of subject and object.[9]

James commented that psychology in his time was hardly more developed than physics had been before Galileo, and despite many advances in the cognitive sciences during the twentieth century, this is still true of the scientific study of consciousness.[10] He added that a topic remains a problem of philosophy only until it has been understood by scientific means, at which point it is taken out of the hands of philosophers.[11] The fact that philosophers continue to make a living by writing book after book claiming to explain consciousness is evidence that the West does not yet have an authentic science of consciousness. Scientists and philosophers continue to speculate on the real nature of the mind, as opposed to its appearances to introspection, by purely logical means, without any compelling empirical evidence. Einstein commented, "Propositions arrived at purely by logical means are completely empty as regards reality. Because Galileo saw this, and particularly because he drummed it into the scientific world, he is the father of modern physics—indeed of modern science altogether."[12]

Philosophy, literally the "love of wisdom," is methodologically aimed at overcoming subjective biases and arriving at theoretical knowledge, which must be a central element of wisdom. Historically, this is the whole point of philosophy. But modern philosophers agree on virtually nothing, and they have produced no body of consensual knowledge, implying that their views must be strongly subject to subjective biases, which detracts from the cultivation of wisdom. The primary reason for this failure is that philosophers have become overspecialized and disengaged from practical philosophy. As ingenious as many of their speculations are, they are commonly of little use either in the world of science or in everyday life.

Most twentieth-century behaviorists, analytical philosophers, and neuroscientists shared two characteristics in their approach to the mind: they assumed that consciousness is a physical function of the body, and they devised no rigorous means of observing consciousness itself. In this they are similar to the scholastic philosophers at the time of Galileo, who refused to question the assumptions of Aristotelian metaphysics and devised no rigorous means of observing the stars or planets. As philosopher Daniel Dennett points out, introspection and consciousness itself are features of the mind that are most resistant to absorption into the mechanistic picture of science.[13] And he adds with striking candor, "With consciousness . . . we are still in a terrible muddle. Consciousness stands alone today as a topic that often leaves even the most sophisticated thinkers tongue-tied and confused."[14]

Some philosophers claim that neuroscientists and behaviorists *indirectly* observe mental events by *directly* observing brain functions and behavior that are related to the mind. If that were true, on the basis of their physical observations, they should be able to tell what the mental events are that they are indirectly observing, without relying on first-person reports of subjective experiences. But they can do nothing of the kind. Without such reports based on the direct experience of the mind, they wouldn't even know that mental events occur, let alone know what they are or what they are about. This fact undermines the widespread and virtually unchallenged notion that mental events are emergent properties of configurations of neurons, similar to the way a wide range of physical properties emerge from other, more basic physical processes.

One remarkable American philosopher who may have foreseen the confusion about consciousness that characterized twentieth-century scientific and philosophical investigations of the mind was Franklin Merrell-Wolff (1887–1985). After graduating from Stanford University with a degree in mathematics and minors in philosophy and psychology, then studying philosophy at Harvard University, and later teaching mathematics at Stanford, he left a promising career in academia to try to fathom the nature of consciousness for himself. His efforts led to a series of remarkable contemplative discoveries in 1936, when he was forty-nine, the effects of which persisted to some extent until his death in 1985. His contemplative inquiries were inspired in part by the Western philosophical tradition, especially Immanuel Kant, and in part by the writings of the Indian contemplative Shankara (mid-eighth century), who first consolidated the views of the Advaita Vedanta school of Hindu philosophy.[15]

Followers of Shankara assert that when we experience an object, this cognition is always accompanied by an immediate self-awareness of the awareness itself. For example, when we see an object such as a pitcher, there simultaneously occurs an awareness of that visual perception. This is called "the witness-consciousness"; it illuminates all phenomena and is infallible, neutral, and eternal, existing independently of anything outside itself.[16] After devoting himself to probing the nature of consciousness by means of such self-awareness, Merrell-Wolff had an insight that he believed played a vital part in clearing the way for the illumination that occurred later. With this insight he realized that so-called empty space was in fact full and substantial, while ponderable objects were a kind of "partial vacuum." Consequently, he began to experience empty space as the substantial foreground while physical objects faded into irrelevancy. This, in turn, led to the perception of material objects as part of a "dependent or derivative reality."[17]

In his initial spiritual awakening, which occurred a few days after this insight, Merrell-Wolff reversed the outward flow of consciousness so that it returned toward its source without projecting an object in the mind, no matter how subtle.[18] This inversion of consciousness, he reported, occurs at the moment of shifting from ordinary dualistic consciousness to a transcendent state, which he experienced as the ground of being. In this shift, he reported, "one consciousness blacks out and immediately another takes over."[19] In the transcendent state, the dualism between subject and object disappears so that one feels a sense of unity with whatever is experienced. One's own sense of personal identity dissolves into a sense of space without any subject-object distinctions. He experienced a sense of depth, abstraction, and great universality in the thoughts that arose while in that state, beyond which there was an "impenetrable Darkness," which he knew to be the "essence of Light."[20] The lingering effects of this realization were a profound sense of contentment, joy, benevolence, and serenity even in the face of adversity.[21]

Merrell-Wolff described his firsthand experiences of transcendent consciousness in ways that are remarkably similar to the accounts of Christian and Hindu contemplatives over the past millennium. Although their interpretations of their experiences are embedded in their respective worldviews, many of these great contemplatives do appear to have tapped into a subtle ground state of consciousness that has thus far eluded mainstream scientific and philosophical inquiry.

THE BUDDHIST INVERSION OF CONSCIOUSNESS

The meditative practice of inverting consciousness—of turning awareness upon itself—was probably first developed in India long before the time of the Buddha, 2,500 years ago, and it was embraced by the Buddha as well. Among the many techniques he taught for achieving *samadhi,* or highly focused attention, he declared that the cultivation of attention directed toward consciousness itself was the most profound.[22] In such practice it is important to recognize that the awareness is not confined within the skull or even the body, so the Buddha taught that one should attend to consciousness by directing the awareness above, below, and in all directions without limit.[23]

The meditative inversion of consciousness was also adopted in the later Mahayana tradition of Buddhism that flourished throughout India and Central Asia. The eighth-century Indian contemplative Padmasambhava gave practical guidance: "Let awareness itself steadily observe itself. At times, let your mind come to rest in the center of your heart, and evenly leave it there. At times, evenly focus it in the expanse of the sky and leave it there. Thus, by shifting the attention in various, alternating ways, the mind settles in its natural state."[24] As this happens, the physical senses withdraw into mental awareness, so that one becomes oblivious to physical surroundings and even the body, and discursive thoughts and mental images also gradually dissolve into the luminous vacuity of the mind. Although Padmasambhava suggests letting one's awareness rest "in the heart," the Buddhist contemplatives, like the Christian contemplatives mentioned earlier in this chapter, do not mean that consciousness is really located in the physical heart.[25]

The eleventh-century Nepalese Buddhist meditation master Maitripa described this practice as follows:

Sit upon a soft cushion in a solitary, darkened room. Vacantly direct your eyes into the intervening space in front of you. Completely dispense with all thoughts pertaining to the past, future, and present, as well as wholesome, unwholesome, and ethically neutral thoughts. . . . Bring no thoughts to mind. Let the mind, like a cloudless sky, be clear, empty, and evenly free of grasping, and settle your awareness in a state of utter vacuity. By so doing, you will experience a quiescent state of awareness imbued with joy, luminosity, and nonconceptuality. Within that state, note whether you experience any attachment, hatred, clinging, grasping, laxity, or excitation, and recognize the difference between virtues and vices.[26]

This meditation on awareness itself has been commonly practiced by Tibetan Buddhists for over a millennium. Panchen Lozang Chökyi Gyaltsen described it like this:

By generating the force of mindfulness and introspection, relentlessly cut off all thoughts completely as soon as they arise, without letting them proliferate. After you have done so, remain in this state without letting thoughts flow outwards, and immediately relax your inner tension without sacrificing mindfulness or introspection.[27]

His instructions on this practice were inspired by the renowned Tibetan woman contemplative Machik Labkyi Drönma (1062–1150), who taught that one should release one's mind in this state of meditative equipoise by alternately concentrating intensely, then gently releasing the awareness, while maintaining an ongoing flow of mindfulness. Unlike in the practice of observing thoughts, described in chapter 7, in this meditation you immediately cut off thoughts as soon as they arise and let your awareness rest in its own nature. The method is likened to a duel between a swordsman and an archer. The thoughts spontaneously flowing from the mind are like arrows being shot by an archer, and the swordsman's task is to flick them away as soon as they draw near.

In the instructions in the previous chapter, you invert your awareness upon itself, concentrating intensely with each inhalation; and with each exhalation you gently release your awareness while cutting off thoughts as soon as you become aware of them. In this way, involuntary thoughts gradually subside and the mind settles in its natural state. As you settle deeper and deeper in this still, luminous state of consciousness, all memories fade away and your ordinary sense of personal identity disappears. You may have the terrifying sensation that you are dropping into an abyss where you will lose your very identity. If this feeling occurs, simply be aware of the fear without being caught in it. This isn't easy, but it is important to rise to the challenge. As you grow more and more accustomed to the practice, you will see for yourself that there is nothing to fear in that luminous darkness. All that has been lost is your conceptually constructed sense of your own self. This is an artificial construct. As your mind settles in its natural state, the sense of "I am" is gradually dismantled. You have begun to explore the deep space of the mind, using the inner telescope of highly focused, clear samadhi.

SAMADHI, A TELESCOPE FOR THE MIND

With the decline of contemplative inquiry in the West and the rise of modern science, attention was directed away from the inner environment of human awareness and outward to the physical universe. Whereas Christian contemplatives had sought to discover the "kingdom of heaven within," the pioneers of the scientific revolution began to probe the heavens above. And they developed their own kind of "samadhi" for enhancing and refining their observations of the firmament. This was the telescope, first invented by the Dutch, then improved upon by Galileo in 1609. With his first instrument he was able to observe celestial objects with an eightfold magnification, but he continued refining his telescopes until they could enlarge images twenty times. It was a challenge to invent such instruments, and even after he had constructed them, he had trouble steadying them due to his trembling hands and the beating of his heart. In addition, he needed to wipe the lenses repeatedly with a cloth, or else they became fogged by his breath, by humid or foggy air, or even by the vapor that evaporated from his eye, especially when it was warm.[28] But Galileo managed to overcome these obstacles and observe the night sky with unprecedented clarity and precision, leading to one new discovery after another.

Since Galileo's time, the science of astronomy has advanced hand in hand with the development of increasingly powerful telescopes. During 2003 and 2004, the Hubble Space Telescope was used to make a million-second-long photographic exposure, taken over the course of 400 Hubble orbits around

Earth. This deep-space probe revealed the first galaxies to emerge from the so-called "dark ages" of the universe, the time shortly after the big bang. The Hubble telescope was directed to a region of space that appeared almost empty to ground-based telescopes. But with the long exposure of a patch of sky just one-tenth the diameter of the full Moon, scientists were able to observe nearly 10,000 galaxies!

Such extraordinary progress in science and technology has revealed the astonishing ability of the human mind to explore the external natural world of the physical universe. But to explore the internal natural world of the mind, one must build and refine the inner telescope of samadhi. The use of highly refined, stable, focused attention has by no means been confined to the contemplative traditions of India, even though they appear to have made the earliest and greatest advances in this field.

Early Christian contemplatives certainly recognized the need to calm the mind and focus the attention, and they made some progress in this regard. Saint Augustine (354–430), for example, described his experience of focused attention as "a state midway between sleep and death: The soul is rapt in such wise as to be withdrawn from the bodily senses more than in sleep, but less than in death."[29] Regarding the contemplative state that arises from inverting awareness in upon itself, he wrote, "It is what the prophet calls our self before we were born and known by God from all eternity: 'Before I formed you in the womb I knew you' (Jeremiah I:5)." Strongly influenced by the writings of Plato, Augustine was convinced that genuine happiness could not be achieved by a transient joining of the soul with the "changeless light" of the mind of God. Rather, the soul must somehow be irreversibly lifted above the realm of change altogether. As described earlier, despite Augustine's long dedication to spiritual practice, by the end of his life he concluded that contemplation is begun in this life but can be perfected only through death, which is viewed by some Christian contemplatives as the ultimate religious experience. This is a fundamental difference between Christian and Buddhist views regarding the potentials of contemplative practice, for Buddhists have always concluded that the highest states of realization may be achieved in this life, resulting in permanent purification and freedom of the mind.

The belief that the mind can be fully liberated only through death is alien to the contemplative traditions of India, where the development of samadhi began centuries earlier and seems to have reached far higher degrees of subtlety and stability. Long before the time of the Buddha, Indian contemplatives were allegedly able to remain in the deepest states of samadhi for hours or even days on end. On one occasion when the Buddha was asked about the difference between his own teachings and those of earlier contemplatives, he responded by claiming that his predecessors did not fully understand the practice of samadhi.[30] This is probably what he was referring to when he claimed elsewhere to have "awakened to meditative stabilization" (*dhyana*), implying not that he was the first to achieve such an advanced state of samadhi, but that he was the first to fully comprehend both the benefits and the limitations of such experience.[31]

Authentic samadhi, according to the Buddha's teachings, is a highly focused state of awareness in which all one's mental faculties are unified and directed onto one particular object. The Sanskrit noun *samadhi* is related to a verb meaning "to put together" or "to collect," such as when one collects wood to kindle a fire. So *samadhi* literally means to "collect" oneself, in the sense of achieving a composure or unification of the mind.[32] The Buddha repeatedly emphasized the importance of bringing the mind under control in this way, so that one can think only what one wishes to think and can control the mind instead of being controlled by it. In this way one learns to subdue the wandering mind, which is likened to taming a rutting elephant.[33]

Buddhists generally speak of four stages of meditative stabilization, each more rarified than the last. Many Theravada Buddhists believe that the first, most basic meditative stabilization provides a sufficient basis in samadhi to reach the highest states of contemplative insight (*vipashyana*), which fully and irreversibly liberate the mind from all its afflictive tendencies. According to the fifth-century Theravada commentator Buddhaghosa, once the first stabilization has been achieved, samadhi can be sustained "for a whole night and a whole day, just as a healthy man, after rising from his seat, could stand a whole day."[34] While the mind is thus absorbed, with the senses entirely withdrawn, one may still engage in discursive thoughts and logical reasoning if one chooses to do so. But the mind no longer obsessively spews forth one involuntary thought after another, and one does not compulsively identify with them and fall into distraction.

After his enlightenment, the Buddha commented on his own struggles to achieve the first stabilization as he addressed a group of monks who were apparently having similar difficulties. Even one of his foremost disciples, named Moggallana, needed his assistance in order to attain this level of samadhi.[35] Perhaps the most important consequence of achieving the first meditative stabilization is that it frees one from the five hindrances: sensual craving, malice, laxity and dullness, agitation and anxiety, and doubt. The first degree of samadhi temporarily purifies these hindrances while in meditation, though they are irreversibly purified only with the subsequent attainment of contemplative insight. With the achievement of the first stabilization it is also much more difficult for them to contaminate the mind after meditation. Even then, the mind remains "malleable," "workable," and "steady, so that one can easily direct it to seeing things 'as they truly are.'"[36] When things are seen as they truly are by a calm and malleable mind, this vision affects the deeper layers of the mind far beyond a superficial intellectual appreciation, because insights will be able to penetrate those regions and thereby bring about inner change.

The Buddha made it clear that the mind must be freed of these hindrances in order to realize the highest state of spiritual freedom.[37] Although scholars disagree as to the minimum degree of samadhi that is needed as a basis for achieving nirvana, there is evidence in the Buddha's teachings as recorded in the Pali canon that the first meditative stabilization is a necessary prerequisite for attaining enlightenment.[38] The Buddha himself did not draw the subtle distinction between the full achievement of this stage of samadhi and "access concentration" to the first stabilization. But later Theravada and Mahayana contemplatives did, and according to many Mahayana Buddhists, this slightly less stable degree of samadhi is sufficient.[39]

Even with the achievement of access to the first meditative stabilization, commonly known as *shamatha* (meditative quiescence), one can maintain flawless samadhi effortlessly and continuously for at least four hours, though perhaps not for a full day and night. With this degree of stability, one can effortlessly sustain meditative equipoise, free of even the subtlest traces of laxity and excitation. Although this state of mental balance is not permanent, it can be maintained by following a contemplative lifestyle and by keeping one's attention honed through regular practice.

Buddhist and Christian contemplatives have drawn different conclusions regarding the possibility of completely purifying the mind of all passions and afflictions, directly perceiving the ultimate nature of reality, and reaching the perfection of contemplative insight within this lifetime. Almost all Buddhists maintain that these ideals can in principle be realized in this life, however rare such an achievement may be, while most Christians believe these goals can be achieved only in the hereafter. There are many important differences in their views of the nature and extent of the impurities of the mind as well as the nature of God and nirvana. But the above discussion raises the question: might some of those differences be due to the relative achievements in samadhi by Buddhist and Christian contemplatives? If Christians had achieved the same levels of meditative stabilization as those claimed by Buddhists, might they have altered their views about the potentials of contemplative practice in this lifetime? These are questions that can be answered only by developing more advanced stages of samadhi, much as the existence of other galaxies can be explored only with high-powered telescopes. Only in this way can the deep space of consciousness, with all its hidden dimensions, be fully explored.

PROBING THE NATURE OF THE OBSERVER

Settle your body in its natural state, either sitting or lying down, and then, while mindfully attending to the tactile sensations throughout your body, let your respiration settle in its natural rhythm. Breathe effortlessly, as if you were deeply asleep, without intentionally trying to modify your respiration in any way.

With your eyes at least partly open, rest your gaze vacantly in the space in front of you. During the in-breath, draw your awareness in upon itself, illuminating its own nature. During the out-breath, release your awareness, letting go of all thoughts and objects of the mind. As you invert your awareness on the inhalation, there is no point at which you detect a real subject, and when you release your awareness during the exhalation, you let go of all contents of the mind, so there is no object to latch onto. With each inhalation, override the flow of obsessive thoughts and images by drawing your awareness in upon the source of these contents of the mind. And with each exhalation, override the compulsive tendency to identify with involuntary thoughts, emotions, and desires by releasing all the contents of the mind. Throughout the whole course of each in-breath and out-breath, gently sustain the awareness of awareness.

As your mind calms, your breathing will become more and more subtle, and when this happens, disengage your awareness from the breath and rest in the ongoing flow of awareness of awareness. Now direct your attention downward, gently release your mind, and without anything on which to meditate, rest both your body and mind in their natural state. Having nothing on which to meditate, and without any modification or adulteration, rest your awareness without wavering, in its own natural state, its natural limpidity, just as it is. Remain in this luminous state, resting the mind so that it is loose and free.

Then, on occasion, pose the question, "What is the consciousness that is concentrating?" Steadily focus your attention, and then raise this question again. Keep doing that in an alternating fashion. This alternation between raising the question and focusing the attention inward is an effective method for dispelling problems of laxity and lethargy. Whenever you are distracted by a noise or some other sensations from your environment, let that serve as a reminder to bring your wandering mind back to the present moment.[1]

Do this practice for twenty-five minutes; then as you rise from meditation, continue to recognize all appearances for what they are: appearances. Don't objectify anything outside, and don't "subjectify" anything inside. View everything as appearances to awareness, with no absolute objects "out there" or subjects "in here." The appearances to your physical senses do not exist independent of your mind, any more than the reflections in a pool of water exist independent of the water. Your thoughts and mental images are simply reflections on your perception. They too do not "re-present" anything already existing out there, independent of your mind. They are simply the contents of your mind, and nothing else.

Whenever you become upset, recognize that nothing out there is the true source of your distress. Nor is the source of suffering in the pure, luminous nature of your own awareness. The fundamental source of your problems is the delusional tendency to reify subjects and objects, grasping onto them as if they are real and concrete, existing by their own nature.

In all your activities maintain unwavering mindfulness, resting as continually as you can in a state of luminous awareness, without grasping onto the inherent existence of objects or subjects. Remain engaged with reality, mindfully present with the events arising around you in the environment and within your mind, without falling back into obsessive thoughts and compulsive grasping. Live as if you were in a lucid dream (recognizing that you are dreaming while you are dreaming), and experiment with shifting your experience of reality by changing the way you view it. This is the road to freedom.

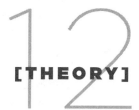

[THEORY]

THE GROUND STATE OF CONSCIOUSNESS

THE GROUND OF BECOMING

According to the earliest accounts of the Buddha's teachings re-corded in the Pali language, he said that by focusing awareness upon its own nature, one eventually apprehends the "sign of the mind." The term "sign" in this context refers to the distinguishing charac-teristics by which one recognizes or remembers something, in this case, the nature of the mind, or consciousness itself.[1] These are the qualities of sheer luminosity and cognizance. In order to identify the defining features of consciousness, not just its neural or behavioral correlates, we must treat it like any other natural phenomenon and observe it directly, with clarity and continuity. Historically, scientific inquiry has been based on objective observation, but conscious-ness cannot be observed objectively or publicly, only in terms of our own subjective experience. As one contemporary philosopher com-ments, the mistake we must avoid is refusing to take consciousness seriously on its own terms. This may require that we "forget about the history of science and get on with producing what may turn out to be a new phase in that history."[2]

This new phase may draw heavily on 2,500 years of experiential inquiry into the nature of consciousness in the Buddhist tradition. When one achieves "access concentration" to the first stabilization, as described in chapter 10, the physical senses become dormant, thoughts and mental images subside, and one's awareness comes to rest in a naturally pure, unencumbered, luminous state known as the *bhavanga,* or "ground of becoming." When you identify this relative ground state of consciousness, you come to know the sign of the mind, or the fundamental characteristic by which the mind can be recognized. This ground state is normally inaccessible, as it mainly occurs during deep sleep, so to unlock the power of the bhavanga, the mind must be fully "woken up" by meditative development, so that its radiant potential may be fully activated.[3]

The bhavanga manifests when awareness is withdrawn from the physical senses and the activities of the mind, such as discursive thoughts and images, have subsided. This happens naturally in dreamless sleep and in the last moment of life.[4] Some early Buddhists regarded the bhavanga as the root consciousness from which all sensory forms of consciousness and mental activities emerge, much as the branches, leaves, and fruit of a tree grow from its root.[5]

THE DEFINING CHARACTERISTICS OF CONSCIOUSNESS

According to many advocates of the Mahayana school of Buddhism, consciousness is characterized by two fundamental qualities: luminosity and cognizance.[6] To get some idea of what is meant by these terms, imagine that you have been immersed in a sensory deprivation tank so efficient that you become entirely unaware of your body and physical environment. Your physical senses pick up nothing. Imagine further that all discursive thoughts, mental images, and other activities of the mind subside. Even in this state of profound inactivity, a kind of vacuity appears to your awareness, and this appearance is produced by the mind's luminous quality. In addition, there is an immediate sense of being aware, and that too is an expression of the mind's luminosity. Consciousness not only *illuminates* this vacuity and its own presence as awareness, it also *knows* that the space of the mind is empty and that there is awareness of that space. That knowing is the cognizance of consciousness, its second defining feature.

Consciousness alone has these two unique qualities. Without it, there are no appearances—no colors, sounds, smells, tastes, tactile sensations, or mental images such as dreams. And without it, nothing is known. When the physical senses are dormant and the activities of the mind are calmed, all that remains is mental awareness, sometimes called introspection. But this term is used in two very different ways: thinking about one's thoughts, emotions, and other mental states and processes, and being aware of the contents of the mind and of awareness itself. Unfortunately, these meanings are often conflated, and this can easily give rise to confusion.

THE SUBSTRATE CONSCIOUSNESS

By engaging in the practice described in the preceding chapter, you may bring previously unconscious memories, fantasies, and emotions of all kinds into the light of awareness. Our common experience of our mental states is heavily edited and processed by the habitual structuring of the mind, so we tend to experience thoughts and emotions that we regard as "normal." But in this training the light of consciousness, like a probe into deep space, illuminates formerly unseen mental processes that seem utterly alien to our past experience and sense of personal identity.

As we consciously expose the deep space of the mind through thousands of hours of observation, we penetrate into normally hidden dimensions that are more chaotic, levels where the order and structure of the human psyche are just beginning to emerge. Strata upon strata of mental processes previously concealed within the subconscious manifest, until finally the mind comes to rest in its natural state, from which both conscious and normally subconscious events arise. This is an exercise in true depth psychology, in which we observe "core samples" of the subconscious mind, cutting across many layers of accumulated conceptual structuring.[7]

The culmination of this meditative process is the experience of the substrate consciousness (*alaya-vijñana*), which is characterized by three essential traits: bliss, luminosity, and nonconceptuality. Bliss does not arise in response to any sensory stimulus, for the physical senses are withdrawn, as if one were deeply asleep. Nor does it arise in dependence upon pleasant thoughts or mental images, for such mental activities have become dormant. Rather, it appears to be an innate quality of the mind when it has settled in its natural state, beyond the disturbing influences of conscious and unconscious mental activity.[8] The luminosity of the substrate consciousness is one of the two defining characteristics of consciousness, and it is that which illuminates all the appearances to the mind. Nonconceptuality in this context is experienced as a deep stillness. But it is not absolutely devoid of thoughts, for this dimension of consciousness is subliminally structured by concepts. When you achieve such attentional balance, you have achieved *shamatha,* and you are able to remain there effortlessly for at least four hours, with your physical senses fully withdrawn and your mental awareness highly stable and alert.

The nineteenth-century Tibetan contemplative Düdjom Lingpa described this process as follows: "Someone with an experience of vacuity and clarity who directs his attention inward may bring a stop to all external appearances and come to a state in which he believes there are no appearances or thoughts. This experience of radiance from which one dares not part is the substrate consciousness."[9] Tibetan contemplatives believe that the experience of the substrate consciousness yields insights into the birth and evolution of the human psyche. Drawing an analogy from modern biology, this may be portrayed as a kind of "stem consciousness." Much as a stem cell differentiates itself in relation to specific biochemical environments, such as a brain or a liver, the substrate consciousness becomes differentiated with respect to specific species. This is the earliest state of consciousness of a human embryo, and it gradually takes on the distinctive characteristics of a specific human psyche as it is conditioned and structured by a wide range of physiological and, later, cultural influences. The substrate consciousness is not inherently human, for it is also the ground state of consciousness of all other sentient creatures. The human mind emerges from this dimension of awareness, which is prior to and more fundamental than the human, conceptual duality of mind and matter.[10] Both the mind and all experiences of matter are said to come from this luminous space, which is undifferentiated in terms of any distinct sense of subject and object. So the hypothesis of the substrate consciousness rejects both Cartesian dualism, as explained earlier, and the belief that the universe is exclusively physical. Moreover, it may be put to the test of experience, regardless of one's ideological commitments and theoretical assumptions.

A contemplative may deliberately probe this dimension of consciousness through the practice described previously, in which discursive thoughts become dormant and all appearances of oneself, others, one's body, and one's environment vanish. At this point, as in sleeping and dying, the mind is drawn inward and the physical senses become dormant. What remains is a state of radiant, clear consciousness that is the basis for the emergence of all appearances to an individual's mind stream. All phenomena appearing to sensory and mental perception are imbued with this clarity and appear to this empty, luminous substrate consciousness.

Although Buddhism is commonly characterized as refuting the existence of a soul, this description of the substrate consciousness may sound as if the concept of a soul is being reintroduced. Whether or not this is the case depends on how you define the soul. The type of self, or soul, refuted in early Buddhism is characterized as unchanging, unitary, and independent. The substrate consciousness, as described in the Great Perfection tradition of Tibetan Buddhism, consists of a stream of arising and passing moments of consciousness, so it is not unchanging or unitary. Furthermore, it is conditioned by various influences, including preceding moments of awareness within the continuum of the substrate consciousness, so it is not independent. Nor is this dimension of consciousness specifically human; rather, it is the subtle continuum of awareness out of which the human mind emerges during the formation of the embryo and into which the mind dissolves during the dying process. Each time you fall into dreamless sleep, your mind dissolves into the substrate consciousness, which is repeatedly aroused into creating one dream after another, each of which dissolves back into this ground awareness, until eventually you awaken and your waking mind reemerges.

When you first experience this blissful, luminous, conceptually silent state, you may easily conclude that this is nirvana or the ultimate nature of consciousness. But Tibetan contemplatives have been insisting for centuries that it is simply the relative ground state of awareness and experiencing it brings about no permanent liberation of the mind. Panchen Lozang Chökyi Gyaltsen, for instance, comments that the experience of this dimension of consciousness enables one to recognize the phenomenal nature of the mind.[11] Düdjom Lingpa likewise asserts that this experience provides insight into the relative nature of the mind, which is not to be confused with the "clear light awareness" or any other exalted state of realization. Indeed, if you get stuck there, advancing no further in your meditative practice, it will not bring you one step closer to enlightenment.[12]

Understandably, modern scientists have not yet replicated this discovery. As long as methods of investigating the mind are limited to the materialistic approaches of studying the brain and behavior, our understanding of the mind will necessarily be materialistic. And the deeper dimensions of consciousness that become evident only with the achievement of inwardly directed *samadhi* will remain unexplored and unknown. For the materialistic scientist, the existence of the substrate consciousness belongs to the realm of metaphysics. However, for the contemplative adept, it is an empirical fact that can be discovered only with highly refined, stable, vivid attention directed, like a powerful telescope, to the inner space of the mind.

THE SUBSTRATE

When one's mind has settled in its natural state, the empty space of which one is aware is called the substrate (*alaya*).[13] Describing it is difficult because, at this point, due to the relative absence of thoughts of "I" and "not I," there is no distinct experience of a division between subject and object. You now have a "subjective" awareness of the substrate that appears as your object—a kind of vacuum into which all mental contents have temporarily subsided. The mind may now be likened to a luminously transparent snow globe in which all the agitated particles of mental activities have come to rest.

The substrate is permeated with a field of creative energy known in the Mahayana tradition as the *jiva,* or life force. This energetic continuum, rather than the brain, is considered to be the actual repository of memories, mental traits, behavioral patterns, and even physical marks from one life to the next.[14] All sensory and mental appearances emerge from the space of the substrate, and it has the capacity to generate alternative realities, such as dreamscapes while asleep. When the substrate manifests in dreamless sleep, it is generally unobservable, and its existence can be inferred only on the basis of waking experience. But with thousands of hours of continuous training in developing mental and physical relaxation, together with attentional stability and vividness, it is said that one may directly, vividly ascertain this inner space and observe how mental and sensory phenomena emerge from it in dependence upon a wide range of psychological and physical influences. When the mind of a contemplatively untrained person dissolves into the substrate at death, the person experiences a brief state of oblivion. But a person who has become familiar with the substrate by probing it with samadhi may cross the threshold of death consciously, vividly recognize the substrate for what it is, and thereby die lucidly. Düdjom Lingpa writes in this regard, "The true substrate is something immaterial, devoid of thought, a space-like vacuity and blankness in which appearances are suspended. Know that you come to that state in deep, dreamless sleep, when you faint, and when you are dead."[15]

By carefully examining the substrate with highly focused, sustained attention, one discovers a kind of relativity of space-time pertaining to the observer and the contents of the mind. You begin by examining the "space" between thoughts, which is characterized by the passage of time. That is, the time between mental events is inseparable from the space between them. You may then determine on the basis of your own experience whether this subjective space-time is constant or changes in relation to the flow of contents of the mind. Does the continuum contract and, expand, or remain the same when thoughts arise? For example, does the space of your mind seem to collapse into thoughts, and does time seem to pass more slowly? If the thoughts have a strong emotional charge, do they influence the space-time of the mind more than thoughts that are emotionally neutral? Do positive thoughts and emotions affect this space-time differently from negative ones, and if so, how?

As you attend to the space of the mind, thoughts and images arise like streams of particles emerging from a vacuum. Fields of positive, negative, and neutral emotions pervade this space, fluctuating from moment to moment, and waves of desire may sweep through, often embedded with thoughts and emotions. The core practice is to observe the arising and passing of all these events, as well as that space-time continuum itself, without letting your awareness collapse.

The Dalai Lama comments on this relativity of space-time,

If you empower your mind by various contemplative practices, a certain realm of reality arises through the maturation of your contemplative insight. Take the example discussed in some Buddhist texts of how meditators in highly evolved states are able to experience eons shrunk into a single instant of time, and also are able to stretch a single instant of time into an eon. From a third person's point of view, what the meditator experiences as an eon is seen only as a single instant. The phenomenon is subjective, unique to the meditator alone.[16]

THE CONSERVATION OF CONSCIOUSNESS

The unified dimension of the substrate and substrate consciousness is neither physical space nor the human psyche. Yet all our experiences of objective and subjective phenomena arise from this stratum, and it provides a portal to a subtler dimension of existence at a more fundamental level than our dualistic world of mind and matter.[17] Contemplatives who have explored this immaterial dimension of reality have discovered a principle of conservation of consciousness that manifests in every moment of experience. No constituents of the body—in the brain or elsewhere—transform into mental states and processes. Such subjective experiences do not emerge from the body, but neither do they emerge from nothing. Rather, all objective mental appearances arise from the substrate, and all subjective mental states and processes arise from the substrate consciousness. In the course of a human life, these mental events are conditioned by the brain and environment, and in turn, they influence the brain, body, and physical environment. But they do not *transform into* those physical phenomena. So contemporary speculations by scientists and philosophers about how the brain produces subjective mental experiences are, from this viewpoint, all based on an unquestioned false assumption: that the brain is solely responsible for the generation of all possible states of consciousness. The explanatory gap in trying to understand how some kinds of neural activity can be equivalent to mental events is unbridgeable, for neural and mental events are never identical.[18]

This view is consistent with the hypotheses of Pythagoras, Socrates, Origen, Saint Augustine, and William James, and it is compatible with everything that is currently known about mind-brain interactions. What Buddhism brings to this confrontation between materialistic and contemplative worldviews is a practical way to test this view by first-person experience, namely through the refinement of the attention and the settling of the mind, especially in the samadhi practice of inverting awareness.

William James proposed three different models to account for the correlations between brain processes and subjective experience: the brain produces thoughts, as an electric circuit produces light; the brain releases, or permits, mental events, as the trigger of a crossbow releases an arrow by removing the obstacle that holds the string; and the brain transmits thoughts as a prism transmits light, thereby producing a surprising spectrum of colors.[19] According to the third model, which is the one James advocated, the stream of consciousness may be a different type of phenomenon than the brain that interacts with the brain while we are alive, absorbs and retains the identity, personality, and memories constitutive in this interaction, and can continue without the brain. Contemporary scientific knowledge of the interactions of the mind and brain is compatible with all three hypotheses proposed by James. But neuroscientists, having no experimental methods for investigating this theory, have simply assumed the validity of the first hypothesis, which accords with their materialistic assumptions, which they virtually never question. Buddhist contemplatives have not been constrained by the ideological commitments of materialism. By subjecting consciousness to the most rigorous, experiential scrutiny, they have made discoveries that challenge some of the most fundamental assumptions underlying modern science.

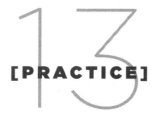

[PRACTICE]

OSCILLATING AWARENESS

Settle your body in its natural state, imbued with the qualities of relaxation, stillness, and vigilance. Then, while mindfully attending to the sensations throughout your body, let your breathing settle in its natural rhythm, breathing as effortlessly as if you were fast asleep.

With your eyes at least partly open and your gaze resting vacantly in the space in front of you, alternate between drawing your attention inward upon yourself as the observer and releasing your awareness into space, not focusing on any object. Follow that by alternating between releasing your awareness and focusing inwardly on that which is controlling the mind, rhythmically releasing and concentration the attention. Pose the question, "What is the agent that releases and concentrates the mind?" Steadily focus your attention upon yourself, then release again. Continue alternating between firmly concentrating your awareness without wavering and gently releasing it, evenly resting it in a state of openness.

14
[THEORY]

CONSCIOUSNESS WITHOUT
BEGINNING OR END

DEATH AND BEYOND

In the modern world, the fate of individual consciousness at death is widely considered to be a matter of religious faith or metaphysical belief. Alternatively, materialists consider the question already answered beyond reasonable doubt: death must entail the termination of individual existence and consciousness. But since scientists—many of whom embrace materialistic views—have not yet identified the necessary and sufficient causes of consciousness, they are equally ignorant of the fate of consciousness at death. Although they are expressing a belief based on inconclusive evidence, many hold to that belief with all the unquestioning tenacity of the most hardcore religious believers. This is a consequence of drawing conclusions about consciousness without having any means of probing its nature directly.

The belief that human consciousness, or the soul, is dispersed and destroyed at death was common during the time of Socrates.[1] However, drawing on the contemplative insights of the Pythagoreans, Socrates himself declared that the truth of what happens at death—contrary to the popular belief in personal annihilation—is known only to those who have studied philosophy. The true philosopher, in his account, "practices death" by shunning sensual craving and corporeal desires. When such a truth-seeker perishes, his soul "departs to a place which is, like itself, invisible, divine, immortal, and wise, where, on its arrival, happiness awaits it, and release from . . . all . . . human evils."[2] But the souls of ordinary people who have not engaged in such philosophical training wander around as spirits after death. Eventually, "through craving for the corporeal, which unceasingly pursues them, they are imprisoned once more in a body. And as you might expect, they are attached to the same sort of character or nature which they have developed during life."[3]

Like the Pythagoreans, the early Hindu contemplatives in India explored the nature and destiny of consciousness with the power of *samadhi*. They reported that at death a stream of individual consciousness, unified with a continuum of vital energy, leaves the body. This stream of consciousness-energy eventually becomes reembodied, over and over again.[4]

The existence of such a life force (*jiva*) that accompanies the subtle stream of consciousness throughout the course of a life and beyond is also asserted in early Buddhist writings. According to one account, a materialist named Prince Payasi ran a gruesome experiment of imprisoning a criminal in a sealed jar until he died, then examined whether there was any objective evidence of his life force leaving the jar when it was opened. When he saw no such evidence, he concluded that no such thing as a life force existed. But the Buddha's renowned disciple Mahakassapa countered that since no such life force entering or leaving a person could be objectively measured when the person dreams, it was unreasonable to expect to see objective evidence of such a force entering or leaving when he dies.[5] Mahakassapa did not refute the prince's hypothesis, only the premise that it could be measured objectively. Like consciousness itself, the life force is something that can be detected only in terms of one's own subjective experience.

Elsewhere in the Pali canon are references to a mind-made body that survives death and has form, including limbs and parts. Even while one is alive, it can be meditatively drawn forth from and return to the coarse physical body. The life force is partly dependent upon the body, but it can leave by means of the mind-made body, which occupies space but does not impinge upon matter. The coarse mind, in contrast, arises together with the formation of the fetus and is dependent upon the physical body.[6]

We noted in chapter 12 that the last moment of the dying process occurs when the coarse mind has entirely and irreversibly dissolved into the ground of becoming, or the substrate consciousness. Immediately before that final dissolution, it is said that there arises a memory of a deed—either wholesome or unwholesome, depending on one's general tendencies throughout the course of life—that indicates the kind of rebirth that lies ahead.[7] Buddhist, Hindu, and Pythagorean contemplatives all concur that the impetus behind this transmigration of consciousness is craving. The Buddha declared that just as a wildfire may be carried far away by the wind, so consciousness is propelled from one life to the next by the current of craving. This impetus continues during the interval after one "lays aside" the body at death and arises in a new body, like a fire carried by the wind across a gap.[8] The interval is called "becoming,"[9] so it naturally follows that the ground of becoming is equivalent to the subtle continuum of consciousness that carries on from one life to the next. It is from this that each individual psyche, or coarse mind, emerges in conjunction with the formation of a physical body.

Early Buddhist texts characterize the intermediate period following death and prior to one's next embodiment as a three-phased period of "wandering and wavering" and "coming and going," during which beings are "seeking to be."[10] The first phase consists of leaving the body with a desire for a further rebirth, like a man leaving a house or a fragment flying off a hot, beaten piece of iron. The second phase is one of wandering back and forth seeking a rebirth, like a man wandering on a road or between houses or a hot iron fragment flying up in the air. The third phase entails falling from one's previous state into a new rebirth, like a man settling down in a square or entering a house or a hot iron fragment falling and cutting into the earth.[11]

JEWISH AND CHRISTIAN VIEWS ON REBIRTH

Belief in rebirth is usually associated with Eastern religions, and it is indeed especially prevalent in those cultures that have developed sophisticated means of refining attention and directing it inward upon the nature of consciousness. Although modern Westerners have failed to devise any such means for probing the depths of consciousness, a remarkable number of Christians and non-Christians believe in rebirth today. According to a Harris Poll taken in 1998, 23 percent of the American public professed belief in reincarnation, including 22 percent of Christians and 32 percent of non-Christians.[12] Similar surveys recently taken in the United Kingdom indicate that 30 to 35 percent of the British population believes in reincarnation.

Although this belief is not accepted in most Jewish and Christian churches today, it is not without basis in the Bible and later theological writings. The first-century Jewish historian Flavius Josephus, for instance, stated that the Pharisees, the Jewish sect that founded rabbinic Judaism, believed in reincarnation. They were the rabbis of the Talmud, who engaged in legal debates about the Torah, but they also practiced forms of meditation. In his account, the Pharisees believed the souls of evil men are punished after death and the souls of good men transmigrate into other bodies, in which they have power to revive and live again. Only the Sadducees, members of another Jewish sect who believed that everything ended with death, did not accept the idea of reincarnation.[13]

One Pharisee cited in the New Testament is Nicodemus, a member of the Jewish ruling council. He once approached Jesus with great reverence, referring to him as "a teacher who has come from God." Jesus replied, "I tell you the truth, no one can see the kingdom of God unless he is born again."[14] Despite Flavius Josephus's assertion that the Pharisees literally believed in reincarnation, it appears that Nicodemus was skeptical on this point, for he asked, "How can a man be born when he is old? Surely he cannot enter a second time into his mother's womb to be born!" Jesus then spoke of the spiritual rebirth that must take place in order to enter the kingdom of God. But he did not refute the possibility of actually being reborn again in the flesh.

Although Christian theologians today generally refute the notion of reincarnation, there is at least one reference to the reembodiment of an individual in the New Testament, cited in chapter 2. This is the prophet Elijah, whom Jesus declared to have been reborn as John the Baptist.[15] The most important Christian theologian to adopt this belief was Origen (185–254). Since there is no account in the scriptures of what preceded the creation of an individual soul, Origen turned to the writings of Plato for answers and claimed that during the beginningless cycles of evolution of the universe, each soul has neither a beginning nor an end. While the physical body wastes away and returns to dust, the immaterial soul is resurrected or reembodied, strengthened by the victories or weakened by the defeats of previous lives.[16] Ultimately, by allowing the wisdom and light of God to shine in this life through the inspiration of Jesus Christ, the individual soul will leave behind the burden of the body and regain complete reconciliation with God.

Unlike many contemporary Christian theologians who believe that God condemns most of humanity and all non-Christians to eternal damnation, Origen maintained that the extent and power of God's love are so great that eventually all things will be restored to him, even Satan and his legions. All men are the "blood brothers" of God himself and cannot remain separated from him forever. Even those who defect must eventually be brought back, and then all things will be made subject to God and God will be "all in all."[17] Origen cited Ephesians 1:4 as evidence for the preexistence of souls: "He chose us in him before the foundation of the world, that we should be holy and without blemish in his sight and love." At the Council of Nicaea in 325, the teachings of Origen were excluded from the doctrines of the Christian Church and fifteen anathemas were proposed against Origen himself. In the council, those advocating Origen's teachings on reincarnation lost by only one vote.

Saint Augustine (354–430), who remains one of the central pillars of Roman Catholic and Protestant theology to this day, proposed four hypotheses regarding the origins of the human soul: it derives from the souls of one's parents; it is newly created from individual conditions at the time of conception; it exists elsewhere and is sent by God to inhabit a human body; and it descends to the level of human existence by its own choice.[18] He found each of these hypotheses to be compatible with the Christian faith, and he declared that one should decide among them only on the basis of sound reasoning.[19]

However, in 543, instead of deciding this issue on the basis of contemplative insight and rational analysis, the Emperor Justinian composed a dogmatic tract proposing nine anathemas against *On First Principles*, Origen's chief theological work. In the same year, he ordered the Christian patriarch Mennas to call together all the bishops present in Constantinople and force them to subscribe to his views. Consequently, the writings of Origen were officially condemned in the Second Council of Constantinople in 553, when fifteen anathemas were charged against him, including the declaration that belief in reembodiment was a heresy. This left open the question of what happens after death. Many Christians now adhere to the conclusion of the Council of Lyons in 1274, which decreed that after death the soul goes immediately either to heaven or to hell. On the Day of Judgment all souls, along with their bodies, will stand before the tribunal of Christ to render account of what they have done. This position was reaffirmed by the Council of Florence of 1439, which used almost the same wording to describe the swift passage of the soul either to heaven or to hell. But this runs counter to the belief of many Christians today that the soul remains in a state akin to deep sleep until the final Day of Judgment, when people will rise up from the grave and meet their maker. Clearly, there has been no consensus on these issues among Christians in the past or today.

Rather than rely on either empirical evidence or cogent reasoning about the origins of the human soul, the Christian Church seems to have left this question to politicians and church councils. Despite the silence of the Bible on this matter, most mainstream Christian theologians since the sixth century have been closed to the possibility of reincarnation. Rather than regarding the question simply as a matter of religious faith, with little or no scriptural basis, it may be more in the spirit of Augustine to investigate it with an open mind.

In Hebrew literature the idea of reincarnation seems to appear for the first time in the writings of Anan teen David (eighth century), who used the term *gilgul* to refer to the transmigration of souls. Within Judaism belief in reincarnation is closely associate with the esoteric tradition known as the Kabbalah. The earliest documented Kabbalistic writing is called the *Book of Formation* (*Sepher Yetzirah*), which, according to one tradition, was written down by the prophet Abraham (c. 1700 B.C.E.), placed in a cave, and then discovered in the first century by Rabbi Shimon Bar Yochai, who was given divine permission to reveal these teachings to his disciples. In the fourteenth century, the Spanish Kabbalist Moses De Leon first presented the *Zohar*, an extremely influential book in Kabbalistic philosophy, which he claimed to have found as scrolls written more than a thousand years earlier. Within this tradition of Judaism, the primary text that describes the complex laws of reincarnation is *The Gate of Reincarnations* (*Sha'ar Ha'Gilgulim*), based on the writings of the master Kabbalist Rabbi Isaac Luria (1534–72) and compiled by his disciple, Rabbi Chaim Vital. *The Book of Splendor* (*Sepher ha Zohar*) gives a rationale for reincarnation that is virtually identical to that of the early Christian theologian Origen. According to this classic of Jewish mysticism, souls must finally reenter the Absolute, whence they emerged. But to accomplish this they must develop the perfections, the seed of which is planted in them. If they have not perfected the virtues by the end of life, then they must reincarnate until all the conditions are met for them to be reunited with God.[20] This belief continues to this day within the Hasidic tradition of Judaism.

BUDDHIST VIEWS ON REBIRTH

Belief in reincarnation is prevalent in all schools of Buddhism, initially stemming from the Buddha's experience of enlightenment. He concluded that three things are necessary for the emergence of a human psyche and the formation of a human embryo: the parents' sexual intercourse; ovulation in the mother; the presence of a being in the intermediate state who has the karma to be reborn to those parents at that time.[21] While such beings are certainly influenced by their karma, or actions in their past lives, they also choose the parents to whom they shall be reborn. So reincarnation is not a matter of predetermination where the future is totally determined by past events.

This contemplative discovery of the existence of past lives has allegedly been replicated by many generations of Buddhist meditators who have developed samadhi and used it to explore the nature and origins of consciousness. This is done primarily through the cultivation of "mindfulness," which has the primary connotation of recollection.[22] Virtually all schools of Buddhism today accept this finding. Although some modern followers of Zen dismiss the Buddhist theory of reincarnation as false or irrelevant, this was not the position of Dogen Zenji (1200–53), the founder of the Soto school of Zen in Japan. A couple of the texts in his principal anthology, *Treasury of the Eye of the True Dharma* (*Shobogenzo*), explicitly deal with the topic. These include *Deep Faith in Cause and Effect* (*Jinshin inga*), which criticizes Zen masters who deny karma, and *Karma of the Three Times* (*Sanji go*), which goes into more detail on the matter.[23]

Most Christians nowadays assume that the soul is newly created from individual conditions at the time of conception, though this is nowhere stated in the Bible, and their common belief is that after death the soul sooner or later goes either to heaven or to hell, never to return. Neither of these beliefs lends itself to empirical or logical verification or repudiation, so they cannot be regarded as scientific hypotheses or philosophical conclusions. They are simply articles of religious faith, without any universally accepted scriptural basis.

SCIENTIFIC STUDIES OF REBIRTH

Most contemporary neuroscientists, psychologists, and philosophers are convinced that the human mind develops together with the formation of the brain and nervous system during gestation and that all mental processes and states of consciousness cease with brain death. In this view, all states of consciousness and all kinds of mental processes are nothing more than functions or emergent properties of the brain. However, as long as study of the mind is confined to investigations of the brain, behavior, and the operations of the ordinary human psyche, knowledge of consciousness will be limited to the operations of the coarse mind, known by way of their physical correlates. The materialistic limitations of this approach predetermine that the resulting view of the mind will be materialistic.

To review: although the assertion that the mind is a physical property of the brain is almost universally accepted among cognitive scientists today, it is not a hypothesis that can be verified or repudiated with the methods of mainstream psychology or neuroscience. It is known that functions of the ordinary mind are closely correlated to specific brain functions, but no one yet knows the exact nature of those correlations. Scientists also remain in the dark concerning the real nature of mental phenomena themselves, and as mentioned earlier, they do not know the necessary and sufficient causes of consciousness in human beings or any other living organism.

Scientific resistance even to considering possible evidence in support of the theory of reincarnation is deeply rooted and fiercely defended, and for good reason. If individual consciousness does not originate from the brain and cease at death, the implications go far beyond scientific understanding of the mind alone. Reincarnation, if true, would imply that the emergence of life and conscious organisms on earth did not occur solely due to material causes. So the theory of evolution would have to be reevaluated from the ground up, taking into account nonphysical influences both in the origins of life and consciousness and throughout the course of biological evolution. And the ramifications would not stop at biology. If nonphysical continua of consciousness carry on from one lifetime to the next, influencing and being influenced by physical organisms, physicists would have to reevaluate the nature of physical causation in the universe at large. Nature would then be seen as open to nonphysical influences, which would allow for spiritual interventions of the kinds theists have been advocating—and materialists have been denying—for centuries. The stakes are indeed high, for the reputations of thousands of scientists and their host institutions are rooted in a thoroughly materialistic view of the universe, and many would feel embarrassment and humiliation if their fundamental assumptions about nature proved to be false. For many, it is safer simply to disregard any empirical evidence that challenges those assumptions. But such imaginary safety based on ignore-ance is contrary to the entire spirit of open-minded, self-critical scientific inquiry.[24] Ironically, scientists who succumb to such closed-mindedness are emulating the medieval scholastics who opposed the birth of modern science. They now stand in the way of unbiased scientific inquiry into the nature of the mind and consciousness much as medieval scholastics stood in the way of scientific inquiry into the nature of the objective physical world.

While Christian and materialist beliefs regarding what happens at death remain largely unquestioned within their respective communities, theories of reincarnation do lend themselves to experiential investigation and rational analysis. Over the past forty years, scientists have identified and studied several thousand cases of young children from all over the world who have accurately reported alleged memories of their past lives. The late Ian Stevenson, professor emeritus of psychiatry and the former director of the Division of Personality Studies at the University of Virginia, pioneered this line of research and wrote extensively on it.[25] His colleague Jim Tucker continues this work in the best spirit of open-minded scientific investigation.[26]

Many people have a hard time remembering even the previous night's dreams when they wake up in the morning, for an automatic forgetting often kicks in immediately as we engage with the sensory experiences and thoughts of the new day. Likewise, memories of a previous life seem to get progressively overlaid by the learning of an infant in its new life. However, if the previous life was suddenly cut short by a violent death, this forgetting process sometimes gets interrupted or delayed. It is as if a sudden death, often occurring relatively early, has left some "unfinished business" that is somehow conducive to remembering details of the previous life. Most of the children with alleged past-life memories Stevenson and his colleagues have studied did report that they had died a sudden and violent death in their previous life. And such children usually stopped speaking about the memories between the ages of five and eight.

It is astonishing to read these accounts of children accurately reporting details of a deceased person's life that they claim as their own past life. Even more remarkable are cases, well over two hundred of which have been carefully studied, in which children have a birthmark or birth defect corresponding to a similar mark, usually a fatal wound, on the deceased person of whom they claim to be the reincarnation. A typical case is that of an Indian boy named Hanumant Saxena, born with a large cluster of vividly pigmented birthmarks near the center of his chest. A few weeks before he was conceived, a man in his village had been shot in the chest at close range with a shotgun and almost immediately died. Between the ages of three and five, Hanumant spoke as if he were this man, and Stevenson was able to confirm by means of a postmortem report the close correspondence between the unusual birthmark on the boy and the fatal gunshot wound of the deceased.[27]

In eighteen other cases Stevenson identified birthmarks on children that corresponded to the entry and exit gunshot wounds of deceased people whose lives they recalled. Often a small birthmark corresponded to the entry wound and a larger and more irregularly shaped one appeared at the site of the exit wound.[28] To account for the transference of such marks from one body to the next, Stevenson postulated the existence of a "field" that retains memories and dispositional characteristics of the deceased. He called this hypothetical field a "psychophore."[29]

As noted in the previous section on the substrate, Buddhism long ago accounted for the transference of such memories and physical characteristics by way of the jiva, or life force, which continues from one lifetime to the next. This may be viewed as a field of information, indivisible from the substrate, that is more fundamental than our human, conceptual constructs of "mind" and "matter." And it is from this information-configured space that our experiences of mind and matter emerge, conditioned by our perceptual experiences and the conceptual frameworks in which we are educated. To draw a contemporary analogy, the transmission of the life force from one incarnation to the next may be likened to software being transmitted by wireless Internet connection from one computer to another. As soon as it is downloaded, it conditions and is conditioned by the hardware of its host, just as downloaded software finds its place within the environment of a personal computer. Likewise, as soon as it is embodied, the life force is influenced by the experiences and behavior of the life form with which it has been conjoined. Thus, at conception there is a confluence of the genetic information received by way of the egg and sperm of one's parents and the past-life information received by way of the life force. The interface between the two represents the interface between the scientific theory of evolution and the Buddhist theory of karma.

It is important to note that in Buddhism only conscious beings such as humans and animals, not plants, are imbued with this life force. It carries the imprints from our previous actions from one life to the next, and when such karma ripens, it manifests not only in the kinds of rebirth we take but also in the type of environment in which we are born and the kinds of events we encounter throughout the course of our lives. Because of the profound entanglement between the mind and the objective world each of us inhabits, even natural disasters such as floods and droughts are said to be caused in part by the past karma of the beings who experience such adversities. So, according to Buddhism, they are not inflicted upon the world by God, nor are they caused solely by the mindless, objective laws of nature. Rather, we are cocreators of the worlds we inhabit, as will be explained later in this book.

According to Tibetan Buddhist accounts, another way one may retain memories from one's past life is by developing advanced states of meditative awareness, supported by high degrees of attentional focus and stability. When accomplished Tibetan contemplatives come to the end of their lives, they may die consciously and continue to maintain conscious awareness through the intermediate period after their death and on into their next rebirth. It is common for their colleagues to seek the reincarnations, or *tulkus*, of such adepts, who in many cases are able as young children to remember many details of their past life, including people they knew; and from an early age they often demonstrate a strong inclination and ability for spiritual practice. In some cases, Tibetan lamas have allegedly told their colleagues where they will be reborn and who their parents will be so that their next incarnation can swiftly be identified without a long search.[30] Memories of their past lives commonly fade away as the tulkus mature, but with further spiritual training they often become accomplished contemplatives again in their current life.

Jim Tucker and a colleague have also studied cases of children who allegedly remember an intermediate period between the end of their past life and their birth in the current life. Such children tend to make more readily verified statements about the previous life they claim to remember than do other children who allegedly recall their past life, and they tend to recall more names. An analysis of reports of thirty-five Burmese children with such memories of the period between their lives indicates that such memories can be broken down into three parts: a transitional stage, a stable stage in a particular location, and a return stage involving choosing parents or conception.

The experiences recalled during the transitional stage were often uncomfortable or unpleasant, and they were associated with the previous life. Some children reported that they saw the preparation of their previous body or the funeral or tried to contact their grieving relatives, only to find that they were unable to communicate with the living. One child said that during this period he did not realize he was dead. This transitional stage often ends as the subject is directed by an elder or an old man dressed in white to a place where he or she then stays for most of the remaining intermediate phase.

During the second stage, subjects reported living in a particular location or having a schedule or duties to which they had to attend, and some reported seeing or interacting with other discarnate beings. They reported varying degrees of comfort during this period. During the third stage, some children claimed to recall following their future parents home, apparently on their own initiative, as the parents passed by while performing everyday tasks, such as bathing or returning from work. Others reported being directed to their present parents, often by elders or by the old man figure referred to in the first stage. These three stages bear some similarity to Buddhist accounts of the three stages of the intermediate period described in the previous section.

While the particular imagery of the intermediate period may be specific to the cultures of those reporting such memories, preliminary study indicates that the three stages seem to be universally applicable. Tucker and his colleague conclude, "Since the children who report such memories tend to make more verified statements about their previous life they claim to remember than do other subjects, and tend to recall more names from that life, their reports of events from the intermission period seem to be part of a pattern of a stronger memory for items preceding their current lives."[31] Instances of children accurately recalling their past lives may be more common worldwide than we might assume, but in a society that rejects the possibility of reincarnation, such alleged memories are naturally dismissed as childhood fantasies.

All case studies of children who allegedly remember their past lives are classified within anthropology, a branch of the social sciences. Given the nature of this research, it was virtually inevitable that it would be ignored or casually dismissed by the scientific community, for there is a very clear hierarchy or pecking order among fields of knowledge within modern academia.

More scientifically compelling evidence comes from the field of "near-death" and "out-of-body" experiences. One of the most remarkable and scientifically noteworthy cases involves the valid out-of-body experiences of a woman undergoing radical brain surgery. In August 1991, Pam Reynolds, a professional singer and songwriter from Atlanta, Georgia, was diagnosed as having an aneurysm in her brain stem, one of the most inaccessible parts of her brain, that could burst at any moment, resulting in death or paralysis. Normally, such a condition was deemed inoperable, but neurosurgeon Robert Spetzler, Director of the Barrow Neurological Institute in Phoenix, Arizona, was an expert at a procedure called hypothermic cardiac standstill, which was the only surgical method that could be used in this situation. In this procedure, the body is cooled down until the heart stops, resulting in clinical death. With the patient's body in a state of suspended animation, surgeons cut the blood flow to the brain to reduce the risk of hemorrhage as they operate.

In Pam's case, a medical team of twenty performed this procedure over a period of six hours and fifty-five minutes. As the surgeons opened up her skull and approached the aneurysm, she was connected to a heart-lung machine that cooled her blood, inducing hypothermia, with her core body temperature dropping below seventy degrees, resulting in her heart stopping except for random quivers of electrical activity. Then the surgeons stopped her heart completely by injecting it with potassium chloride, the same drug used on death row, resulting in her core body temperature dropping to sixty degrees. Her brain stem stopped responding, and the surgeons then drained the blood vessels in her brain, including the aneurysm. After the blood vessel was repaired, the heart-lung machine rewarmed her body until her heart showed signs of life.

The day following her surgery, she reported recollections that began soon after she was anesthetized with a heavy dose of barbiturates, which would have further shut down her brain, resulting in a very deep comatose condition. She recalled that during the operation, she had a sense as if she could feel a suction sensation at the top of her head, and then she was out, looking down at her body, with a great view of everything with crystal-clear vision, even though her eyes were taped shut, and hearing sounds in the room with unprecedented clarity, even though plugs had been inserted in her ears. Looking down, she saw an instrument in Dr. Spetzler's hand with interchangeable bits, and she heard a guttural noise that pitched out as a natural D. She recollected not only the distinct sound of the operating drill but also distinct speech. This included her recollection of a female voice saying, "We have a problem. Her arteries are too small." When she was jolted back to life after the operation, she felt as if she had been dropped into a pool of ice water. When she reported these recollections to her health care providers, they acknowledged that everything she described was accurate. Fifteen years later, she commented that the memory of this experience had remained clear from year to year without fading or becoming foggy.

Dr. Karl Greene, one of the neurosurgeons at the Barrow Neurological Institute, commented with open candor, "When it comes to the whole issue of consciousness and the brain, all bets are off." And Dr. Spetzler remarked, "She really had a sort of bird's-eye view of what was going on. Now whether that image came from somewhere else that she then internalized somehow, I don't think there's any way to tell. But it was sort of intriguing with how well she described what she shouldn't have been able to see." There simply is no scientific—or rather, materialistic—explanation for Pam's out-of-body visual and auditory experiences while her brain was flatlined, with no blood flow. This is one of the clearest clinical cases indicating the limitations of scientific inquiry and explanation as long as scientists insist that the only scientific explanations are ones that accord with the metaphysical assumptions of materialism.[32] Here is what this totem pole of contemporary knowledge looks like:

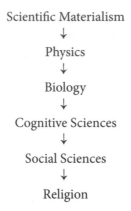

Scientific Materialism
↓
Physics
↓
Biology
↓
Cognitive Sciences
↓
Social Sciences
↓
Religion

An unwritten rule of scientific inquiry is that all research in physics must be conducted in accordance with the principles of scientific materialism. If physicists conduct empirical research into areas that are deemed "paranormal" or "supernatural," they are likely to face strong disapproval. For example, the Nobel Prize-winning physicist Wolfgang Pauli collaborated with Carl Jung in postulating the existence of an archetypal dimension of reality that transcends the bifurcation of mind and matter.[33] Although his ideas are consistent with modern physics, knowing that they violate the principles of scientific materialism, Pauli refused to allow his writings on this subject to be made public until after his death, out of fear of ridicule from his peers. This was same reason Copernicus would not let his heliocentric theory of the solar system be published during his lifetime. He feared condemnation by the Roman Catholic Church, his employer, which could have resulted in his excommunication and eternal damnation.

In line with the above hierarchy, biologists are severely discouraged from engaging in any research or line of inquiry that violates the laws of contemporary physics; cognitive scientists must defer to the current views of biologists; social scientists must confine their inquiries to the beliefs of the cognitive sciences; and secular scholars of religion must view their subject matter in accordance with the methods and views of all other academic disciplines. Ian Stevenson and his colleagues at the University of Virginia, employing methods of the social sciences, have challenged this hierarchy. Their conclusions concerning reincarnation reject some of the core beliefs of the cognitive sciences, which are higher up on the totem pole than the social sciences.

In so doing, they also challenge the materialistic assumptions of biology and physics, and in modern academia, this is simply unacceptable to many scientists. No matter how rigorous their methods or compelling their evidence, they are going against centuries of scientific inertia, a view that has always marginalized the role of consciousness in the natural world, which is still likened to a mindless machine, as Descartes hypothesized at the dawn of modern science.

CONTEMPLATIVE SCIENTIFIC RESEARCH INTO CONSCIOUSNESS

In his advocacy of psychology as a natural science, William James proposed that introspection—the direct observation of mental phenomena—should be the primary means of investigating the mind. Only through introspection could one make refined observations and careful experiments that could provide a wider vision of the nature of the mind and its role in the natural world. He was deeply skeptical of the mechanistic materialism that already dominated all branches of science during his time, so he applied himself most diligently and with the greatest effort in exactly those places where it seemed most likely that the assumptions of materialism might be proven wrong. This led him to take both religious experience and reports of psychic phenomena very seriously, approaching both fields with great intelligence and open-mindedness. Unfortunately, his radically empirical approach to the study of consciousness has been eclipsed over the past century by the methods of generations of behaviorists, psychologists, neuroscientists, and philosophers who have confined their empirical and theoretical inquiries within the metaphysical framework of mechanistic materialism. They have avoided most diligently and with the greatest effort those places where it seemed most likely that their theories might be proven wrong. As a result, this past century has seen virtually no progress in terms of discovering the nature and origins of consciousness in human beings or in the course of evolution as a whole.

The Buddhist tradition, on the contrary, has taken a radically empirical approach to the study of the mind for the past 2,500 years, and Buddhist contemplatives claim to have made many fundamental discoveries about consciousness, including its continuity from one life to the next. As mentioned previously, the Buddha's own experiential insights into the existence of his own and others' past lives have allegedly been replicated thousands of times by Buddhist contemplatives, even in the recent past. The Buddha achieved his realization of past lives through the power of samadhi, and specific instructions for replicating this mode of contemplative inquiry are to be found in Buddhaghosa's classic work, *The Path of Purification*.[34] The contemporary Burmese meditation master Pa-Auk Tawya Sayadaw has also explained how to acquire such past-life recall, as has the late Tibetan Buddhist scholar Geshe Gedün Lodrö.[35] But this kind of research has never been conducted in collaboration with scientists, under controlled conditions.

According to Buddhaghosa, ideally one first achieves the fourth meditative stabilization, a highly advanced stage of samadhi in which the breath ceases altogether and the mind settles in a profound state of equilibrium, with all the physical senses withdrawn into mental awareness. It is claimed that someone who has achieved this can remain in meditation for days on end, entirely oblivious of their surroundings. Given the rarity of this accomplishment, I once asked a senior Tibetan meditation master named Yangthang Rinpoche, renowned among his Tibetan Buddhist peers for profound meditative realizations, whether it is also possible to accurately recall one's past lives on the basis of the more modest achievement of *shamatha*, previously discussed in chapter 10. He replied, "Yes, due to the luminosity of this state of consciousness, extrasensory perception arises spontaneously, and that includes the ability to recall past lives." But, he added, "it's an open question whether people can still achieve shamatha nowadays."[36]

Recognizing the vital role that achievement of shamatha plays in the Buddhist path to liberation, since 2003 I have been collaborating with a team of psychologists and neuroscientists at the University of California, Davis, on a scientific study known as the Shamatha Project.[37] In February 2007, the Santa Barbara Institute for Consciousness Studies and UC Davis began the first phase of this study, in which thirty-seven people gathered at a retreat center in Colorado and practiced shamatha for eight to ten hours each day for three months. During this time they were subjected to a wide range of physiological and psychological measurements by a team of five scientists studying the effects of such intensive meditation over a sustained period of time. In September of that year, a second group of thirty-three people (the control group for the scientific study) embarked on their own three-month retreat. Although only a fraction of the terabytes of data gathered in this study has been analyzed at the time of writing this book, there is clear evidence that this three-month training resulted in a decrease in afflictive attachment, anxiety, difficulties in emotion regulation, and neuroticism, and an increase in mindfulness, conscientiousness, empathic concern, dispositional positive emotions, and general well-being.

More than a year after the conclusion of the first retreat, a dozen of the participants are continuing in full-time practice, meditating up to twelve hours each day, and, as the meditation instructor for the study, I continue to guide them in their practice. As Yangthang Rinpoche commented, it is an open question whether people in the modern world can do this, and as the initiator of the project, I am committed to seeking an answer.

Even with the accomplishment of shamatha, it may take further meditative training before one can accurately recall distant memories. As mentioned in chapter 12, according to many Buddhist contemplatives, memories are stored in the life force, which is of the same nature as the substrate (*alaya*). Once the mind has settled in the substrate consciousness following the achievement of shamatha, it is said that one can direct one's attention to the past, successively targeting specific times in the more and more distant past, even prior to one's birth in this lifetime. This suggests the possibility of a scientific study, which might be called the Alaya Project, to put the Buddhist hypothesis of past lives to the test of experience.

Such a study would require a group of subjects (the larger, the better) to achieve shamatha. While resting in the substrate consciousness, they would focus their attention upon a specific time, beginning perhaps one week earlier to the exact hour and minute. Subjects would focus their attention on this target until they were confident that they had vividly recalled their experiences exactly one week before, and they would give a detailed report of their alleged memories. Then the accuracy of their reports would be checked by objective means, such as questioning other people who were with them at that earlier time. If their memories proved to be valid, they would then target an earlier date, and again the accuracy of the reports would be investigated. This process of directing the attention further and further back in time would continue as long as their reports could be put to the test of objective corroboration.

Eventually, they would be directed to focus their attention to a specific time before they were conceived. If they recalled nothing, this would support the materialists' claim that consciousness originates during the development of the brain. But if they recalled experiences of being someone else in a past life, these alleged memories could be checked objectively to see if they corresponded to real people who lived in the past. One would further need to ascertain whether the subjects had any access to this information by normal means outside of meditation. If their memories proved to be accurate and it could be established beyond all reasonable doubt that they could not otherwise know the details of the lives of the deceased individuals whom they had recalled, this would support the Buddhist hypothesis of rebirth. Such a study would constitute a rigorously scientific way to put the Buddhist theory to the test of experience.

If memories are indeed stored in a continuum that precedes this life, we might well ask, why is it that we do not remember our past lives? Tibetan Buddhism likens the dying process to falling asleep, the intermediate state to dreaming, and conception to waking up. In the course of a single night, people normally experience five to seven dream cycles, beginning about ninety minutes after they fall asleep. When entering the first dream cycle, people normally have forgotten the events of the preceding day, and for the time being, their reality is comprised only of the events in that dream. After some minutes, they fall back into dreamless sleep, during which their minds settle back into the substrate consciousness. In this process, they tend to forget the events of the dream that has just ceased. Then after an hour or two, they enter their second dream cycle, once again oblivious of the events of the day and of their previous dream. This process of repeated amnesia continues throughout the night until they finally emerge from their last dream into the waking state. At this point, some people can clearly recall one or more dreams of the night, but many find it difficult to remember even the dream immediately before waking. And the more they become involved with the events of the day, the less they can usually recall their dreams of the night.[38]

This cycle of amnesia throughout a day and night is said to parallel what goes on from the time that one dies, through the experiences of myriad dreamlike events during the intermediate state, and eventually when one takes rebirth. Plato referred to the lapse of recollection between lives in his account of the myth of Er at the end of *The Republic*, where he declared that the souls of men drink from the waters of forgetfulness as they proceed from one life to another.[39] The Tibetan Buddhist practice of dream yoga is designed to overcome this amnesia during sleep by enabling one to recognize and explore the dream state while dreaming.[40] This is called a lucid dream, and lucid dreamless sleep occurs when one knows that one is in dreamless sleep while it is happening, while one rests in the substrate consciousness. Such training prepares one to recognize the substrate consciousness in the final phase of dying and then to recognize the events of the intermediate state for what they are. With such lucidity, one may wisely direct one's consciousness to the next rebirth in a way that is of benefit to oneself and others. That is the central purpose of dream yoga.

The Alaya Project would approach the hypothesis of rebirth from a psychological perspective, but it is also possible to test the Buddhist theory in terms of biological evidence. Buddhist contemplatives claim that the life force, or jiva, that carries on from one life to the next is "physical" in the sense that it directly influences and is influenced by the body. But the life force is immaterial, for it is not composed of material particles. There are similar instances of physical, immaterial phenomena in modern physics. Electromagnetic fields in classical physics, Hilbert space and probability waves in quantum physics, and space-time in relativity theory are all regarded as physical phenomena, but none of them is composed of atoms or elementary particles. As mentioned previously, the life force is the repository of memories, mental traits, and behavioral patterns. Its configuration is influenced by the physical body, and imprints on the life force influence the formation of the body from life to life.

Ian Stevenson and his colleagues have studied a number of cases in which the manner of death in one lifetime allegedly leaves birthmarks on the body in the next life.[41] The configuration of each person's life force is utterly unique, and it changes over time as it accumulates imprints from ongoing experiences. The life force that conveys the imprints resulting in such birthmarks is closely related to a kind of vital energy (*prana*) said to be located in the center of the chest and in turn closely related to the substrate consciousness. If, by way of the vital energies associated with this life force, there is a direct interface between it and the electromagnetic fields generated in the body, then there should also be a unique signature of the electromagnetic fields for each individual. Moreover, the substrate consciousness most regularly manifests during dreamless sleep, and this would imply that at that time each person may exhibit a unique electroencephalographic signature. Recent scientific studies do indicate evidence for such unique EEG signatures.[42]

This suggests a scientific study that might be called the Jiva Project. In this proposed study, the unique EEG signature of an elderly, highly advanced Tibetan Buddhist contemplative would first be identified. If it was closely correlated with the vital energy configuration of that person's life force, then it would be possible that this signature would carry over into the next lifetime. Since in the Tibetan tradition it is common for the reincarnations of accomplished contemplatives to be sought out and identified as tulkus, after the elderly contemplative had died and his alleged reincarnation had been identified, scientists could then check to see whether the EEG signature of the child and the deceased contemplative matched. If they did, this would provide strong physical evidence of the continuity of the life force from one rebirth to the next.

According to Buddhist theory, what carries on after death is not an unchanging, unitary, independent soul, self, or energy. Rather, it is an ever-changing stream of consciousness and energy that gives rise to the formation of a human psyche and conditions the formation of the embryo during gestation. The very first moment of consciousness in a developing fetus consists of the substrate consciousness alone, and that consciousness is all that is left in the final stage of the dying process. There is a perfect symmetry, with the end of life reflecting the beginning in a cyclic process that constitutes the nature of sentient existence in the universe. In this continuum of consciousness and energy from life to life there is no enduring, immutable self, only a stream of dependently related mind-body events arising in dependence upon prior causes and conditions.

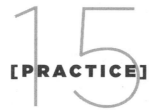

[PRACTICE]

RESTING IN THE STILLNESS OF AWARENESS

Settle your body in its natural state and your breathing in its natural rhythm, and then with your gaze resting vacantly in the space in front of you, steadily focus your attention up into the space above you, without desire and without bringing any object to mind. Relax again. Then steadily, unwaveringly direct your awareness into the space on your right, then on your left, and then downward. In this way, begin to explore the space of awareness, noting whether it has any center or periphery.

At times, let your awareness come to rest in the center of your chest and evenly leave it there. At other times, evenly focus it in the expanse of the sky and leave it there. By shifting your attention in this way, you will allow your mind to gradually settle in its natural state. Following this practice, your awareness will remain evenly, lucidly, and steadily wherever it is placed. Due to the force of the attention being focused single-pointedly inward, the physical senses become dormant, and with the settling down of involuntary thoughts, the mind dissolves into the substrate consciousness. Your consciousness now rests in peace, pervaded by a sense of luminous wakefulness and an even sense of well-being.[1]

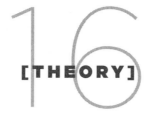

[THEORY]

WORLDS OF SKEPTICISM

SCIENTIFIC SKEPTICISM

The Buddhist hypothesis of a life force that carries over from one physical embodiment to the next is reminiscent of the discredited scientific proposal that living beings are endowed with a life force known as the *élan vital*. Despite the popularity of this view in the nineteenth century, no one was ever able to objectively detect such a life force, and in 1938 the Russian biologist Aleksandr Oparin proposed an alternative theory that life originates from nonlife, implying a smooth continuum from inorganic to organic matter. Scientific acceptance of this hypothesis gained great momentum in 1953 when the American biologist Stanley Miller mixed basic gases approximating the Earth's early atmosphere with an electric charge inside a glass chamber and produced amino acids, a building block of life. Although scientists then appeared to be on the cusp of freshly creating life in the laboratory, all such attempts have failed. In a 1996 Reuters interview Miller acknowledged, "Making the amino acids made it seem like the rest of the steps would be very easy. It's turned out that it's more difficult than I thought it would be. It's a series of little tricks. Once you learn the trick it's very easy. The problem is learning the trick."[1]

An amino acid and a living cell are vastly different entities. In a single cell many thousands of components dynamically interact with one another in very complex ways, and each component depends on the actions of many others. The transformation—or lack of transformation—of one component may affect an entire chain of events, or even the functioning of the whole cell. Amino acids of the kind that Miller created may be likened to single screws, while a living cell can be compared to a functioning watch. Individual screws are certainly useful, for without them you cannot make a watch, just as amino acids are necessary for the formation of a cell; but amino acids on their own are dead and do not interact as do the components of a living cell. So Miller's comment that all that stands between amino acids and a living cell is a "series of little tricks" is like saying that the difference between single screws and a watch is nothing more than a series of little tricks. There is a major difference, though: watchmakers know how to assemble screws and other mechanical components to construct a watch, but biologists have no idea how to artificially create the steps from amino acids to a living organism. Once a replicating organism exists, they know how mutation and natural selection can modify such life to achieve the kinds of diversity we see, but that does not explain the origins of the first single-celled organism.

Oparin's hypothesis has never been validated—no one has yet created a living organism out of inorganic molecules—but it is now widely accepted as an established scientific fact. The origin of life in the universe has been relegated to a "series of little tricks," which the scientific community trusts that future generations will discover and thereby validate their current, materialistic assumptions. Any other hypothesis, such as an élan vital, now seems utterly implausible, for no such vital energy has ever been detected in a scientific laboratory. This is the same reasoning by which radical behaviorists of the 1950s denied the existence of subjective mental states: they don't exist because they cannot be measured scientifically. This absurd belief has been abandoned by most cognitive neuroscientists, who are now intent on discovering the neural correlates of subjective mental states and their behavioral expressions.

Nevertheless, most cognitive scientists still assume that all mental phenomena, including consciousness itself, are emergent properties of the brain interacting with our physical and social environment. Although the mind has not been explained purely in terms of physics and genetics, it is almost universally assumed to exist as a system of physical processes. This is remarkable, for no subjective experience—even one as simple as physical pain—can be measured with any of the instruments of technology, which are capable of detecting all known kinds of physical events. And when subjective mental states are observed introspectively, they exhibit no physical attributes at all: they do not appear to have mass, location or dimensions within physical space, velocity, or any other physical qualities. Even so, most scientists still assume without question that they must be physical attributes of the brain—quite a leap of faith!

Mental states are now commonly likened to computer programs that carry information, but information can be said to be present in computer programs only in relation to conscious programmers who create them and computer users who make sense of them. To illustrate this point: while playing a game of chess with the computer Deep Blue, you may consciously think about your next chess move, while Deep Blue unconsciously calculates its next move. Everything Deep Blue does can be understood in terms of mathematical algorithms, with no reference to consciousness.

There are no logical or empirical grounds for believing that chess moves literally "appear" to Deep Blue or that it consciously "knows" how to play chess. Likewise, there is no good reason to believe that current computer systems are imbued with conscious self-understanding. The workings of computers are thoroughly understood in terms of the current laws of physics, and these mechanical interactions can be made to *simulate* behavior that corresponds to conscious human mental activity. But to jump to the conclusion that such interactions constitute conscious processes is similar to imputing motives, feelings, and desires to weather formations, volcanic eruptions, and earthquakes. This is simply a modern version of animism, expressed, ironically, by many contemporary advocates of artificial intelligence.[2]

Such confusion is especially prevalent in the current field of robotics. Robot learning can be defined as the robot making new versions of its original instructions, collecting and sorting data in a creative way. When a robot unconsciously "learns" something, what it is really doing is integrating the group of simultaneous computer programs with which it began. But when human observers see a robot's eyes move, see its head turn, see the programmed chest motion that looks so much like breathing, they start talking about it as a living thing. Modern, superstitious animism strikes again!

Researchers in this field believe that robot consciousness is related to two areas: robot learning (the ability to think, to reason, to create, to generalize, to improvise) and robot emotion (the ability to feel). Robot learning has already occurred in the sense that the machines are able to learn new skills that go beyond their initial capabilities, but there is no evidence that robots consciously know or understand anything! Some researchers feel that robots will one day be able to experience emotions as well, even though they have no way to test that hypothesis. Rodney Brooks, the former director of MIT's Computer Science and Artificial Intelligence Laboratory, goes so far as to say that robot emotions may already have occurred, that sophisticated robots not only display behavior associated with emotions but also actually experience them. Although there is no empirical evidence to support this faith-based claim, he indirectly justifies it by declaring, "We're all machines. Robots are made of different sorts of components than we are—we are made of biomaterials; they are silicon and steel—but in principle, even human emotions are mechanistic."[3] Instead of supplying any evidence for his belief in robot emotions, he backs it up with another belief, namely that humans are really nothing more than robots! In this way, one unsubstantiated belief is built on another equally unsubstantiated belief, all under the guise of science.

Without questioning the validity of this mechanistic view of consciousness, Brooks overlooks the fact that human emotions are undetectable by any objective physical means and simply asserts that a human emotion like sadness consists of various neurochemicals circulating in the brain. If this is true, he reasons, a robot's level of a feeling like sadness could be set as a number in computer code.

Relying on a metaphysical ideology rather than supporting empirical evidence, he declares, "Humans are made up of biomolecules that interact according to the laws of physics and chemistry. We like to think we're in control, but we're not." This would mean that humans and robots alike, whether made of flesh or of metal, are basically just sociable machines. But Lijin Aryananda, a researcher in the Artificial Intelligence Lab at the University of Zurich, brings us back to the empirical facts unadorned with metaphysical speculation: "Anyone who tells you that in human–robot interactions the robot is doing anything—well, he is just kidding himself. Whatever there is in human–robot interaction is there because the human puts it there."[4] Scientists have not yet found a way of putting consciousness into a robot, and even if they had, they have no way of detecting such consciousness. The obvious reason for that is that they don't even have a way of detecting consciousness in human beings or any other living creature.

The origins of life and of consciousness remain scientific mysteries to this day, despite all the advances in genetics, neuroscience, artificial intelligence, and robotics. The scientific community has not yet agreed upon a definition of consciousness; has no objective, scientific means of measuring it; and does not know the necessary and sufficient causes for the generation of consciousness. William James commented on this level of scientific ignorance about the nature of mental phenomena more than a century ago, and—under the domination of the assumptions of mechanistic materialism—little progress has been made since his time. What has been omitted in all such research over the past century is the first-person perspective of experiencing one's own body-mind. And it is on the basis of centuries of such empirical evidence—rather than a commitment to a metaphysical creed and hope in future scientific breakthroughs—that Buddhist accounts of the life force and the origins of consciousness are made.

The Buddha summarized the spirit of contemplative skepticism with the words:

> Do not go upon what has been acquired by repeated hearing; nor upon tradition; nor upon rumor; nor upon what is in a scripture; nor upon surmise; nor upon an axiom; nor upon specious reasoning; nor upon a bias towards a notion that has been pondered over; nor upon another's seeming ability; nor upon the consideration, "The monk is our teacher." . . . When you yourselves know: "These things are good; these things are not blameable; these things are praised by the wise; undertaken and observed, these things lead to benefit and happiness," enter on and abide in them.[5]

PHILOSOPHICAL SKEPTICISM

With the rise of behaviorism in the early twentieth century, subjective experience in general and consciousness in particular were marginalized due to the insistence that the scientific study of the mind be purely objective. B. F. Skinner (1904–90), the most renowned and influential of all American behaviorists, did not question the practical usefulness of the inner world that is felt and introspectively observed, but he insisted that mental states and processes cannot be clearly observed or known.[6] In fact, he went so far as to declare that no one has ever directly modified any mental activities or traits such as thoughts, opinions, urges, choice, interests, or daydreams, and that there is no way we can make contact with them.[7] This weird claim, so obviously incompatible with everyday experience as well as science, suggests that Skinner had exceptionally limited introspective abilities that severely impaired his understanding of the mind. Rejecting the possibility of defining consciousness in terms of its characteristics as they are experienced firsthand, he chose instead to equate the experience of knowing to a "very special form of behavior."[8] This is a patently false claim, for it is obvious that we can know things before we act on them or without ever acting on them, and human beings and robots alike can engage in unconscious behavior.

From a contemplative perspective, the entire school of behaviorism, for all its valuable insights into human and animal behavior, appears to have been created and developed by individuals who were mentally impaired in terms of their abilities to observe their own subjective experience. It is hardly any wonder then that Skinner and other behaviorists were so intent on characterizing the mind in purely physical terms, first substituting the brain for the mind and then substituting the person for the brain.[9]

While many scientists today regard the principal views of behaviorism as deeply flawed and long rejected, many of those same beliefs are advocated by contemporary analytical philosophers, such as Daniel C. Dennett. In his view of human nature, "*we* are robots made of robots—we're each composed of some few trillion robotic cells, each one as mindless as the molecules they're composed of, but working together in a gigantic team that creates *all the action* that occurs in a conscious agent."[10] Although like Skinner, he acknowledges that each of us has our own introspective experience of our mental states and activities, he insists that we must not credit those intuitions. After all, he points out, although it *appears* that the Sun rotates around the Earth, this perception is misleading, and similar reliance on the introspective appearances of mental events is likewise bound to obscure the real nature of the mind and consciousness. However, if Galileo had not credited his firsthand observations of the Sun, Moon, and planets, enhanced by his use of the telescope, he would never have taken his seminal role in the history of astronomy and science as a whole. But when Dennett considers the potential contributions of Christian and Buddhist contemplatives for understanding the nature and potentials of consciousness, he is simply dismissive: "It seems to me that the best that can be said of them is that they manage to stay out of trouble, which is not nothing."[11]

John R. Searle, another prominent analytical philosopher, summarizes the effects of the twentieth-century marginalization of subjective experience in the scientific and philosophical investigations of consciousness:

> It would be difficult to exaggerate the disastrous effects that the failure to come to terms with the subjectivity of consciousness has had on the philosophical and psychological work of the past half century. In ways that are not at all obvious on the surface, much of the bankruptcy of most work in the philosophy of mind and a great deal of the sterility of academic psychology

over the past fifty years . . . have come from a persistent failure to recognize and come to terms with the fact that the ontology of the mental is an irreducibly first-person ontology.[12]

What he is emphasizing here is that the reality of first-person experience cannot be reduced to anything else, such as behavioral dispositions or the activity of neurons; that is, subjective experience is ontologically irreducible. "Because mental phenomena are essentially connected with consciousness," he writes, "and because consciousness is essentially subjective, it follows that the ontology of the mental is essentially a first-person ontology. . . . The consequence of this . . . is that the first-person point of view is primary."[13] Searle goes on to acknowledge the possibility of "self-consciousness," in which we shift our attention from the object of conscious experience to the experience itself.[14] Ironically, despite his insistence on the primacy of the first-person perspective on mental events, Searle is no more sympathetic to introspection than his fellow philosopher Dennett.[15]

Especially since the 1990s "decade of the brain," a growing number of neuroscientists have begun to focus their research on the neural correlates of a wide range of mental processes. Despite their many successes in discovering connections between specific mental and brain events, the actual nature of mental processes and their relation to the brain remains a mystery. Moreover, no one yet has identified the neural correlates of consciousness itself. B. F. Skinner felt that those who rejected his reduction of mind to behavior had "done a great disservice by leading physiologists on false trials in search of the neural correlates of images, memories, consciousness, and so on."[16] But the Dutch neuroscientist Victor A.F. Lamme recently countered that the trouble began with the insistence that the presence or absence of conscious experience always has to be probed behaviorally. In his view, "we need to let go of our intuitive or psychological notions of conscious experience and let the neuroscience arguments have their way. Only by moving our notion of mind towards that of brain can progress be made."[17]

With a complete rejection of introspection as a means to probe the nature of consciousness, he proposes that recurrent interactions between cortical neurons are the crucial feature of consciousness. By defining consciousness solely in terms of these interactions, he believes, the long-standing debates about consciousness among philosophers and psychologists can be put to rest. But many neuroscientists are skeptical of this reductionist view of the mind, among them Christof Koch, who has devoted a great deal of effort to identifying the neural correlates of consciousness.

Scientists generally define natural phenomena in terms of their observed qualities, but one may know a great deal about recurrent interactions between cortical neurons, yet know nothing about consciousness as it is immediately experienced. And one may know a great deal about one's immediate experience of consciousness without knowing anything about such interactions. So there doesn't seem to be any justification for describing consciousness in terms of brain activity. Doing so is simply a decision to equate something one doesn't understand scientifically with something that one does understand, at least to a better extent.

Lamme has not been able to silence debate on this issue even among his fellow neuroscientists, let alone among philosophers and psychologists, who have come to no consensus about the nature of consciousness. The true spirit of philosophical skepticism is expressed by the Jewish existentialist Martin Buber: "I have occasionally described my standpoint to my friends as the 'narrow ridge.' I wanted by this to express that I did not rest on the broad upland of a system that includes a series of sure statements about the absolute, but on a narrow rocky ridge between the gulfs where there is no sureness of expressible knowledge but the certainty of meeting what remains undisclosed."[18]

CONTEMPLATIVE SKEPTICISM

Scientists often cite this principle for evaluating novel theories and hypotheses: extraordinary claims require extraordinary evidence. One question they almost invariably overlook, however, is: "extraordinary" for whom? If there is only one valid worldview—one absolutely valid perspective on reality—such as that of contemporary science, then the question is quickly answered. In that case, a theory is extraordinary if it goes against the grain of current, mainstream scientific beliefs. But if there are multiple, empirically based perspectives on reality—such as scientific and contemplative views on the nature of consciousness—then a theory that may be "extraordinary" for one community may be commonplace for another.

Take, for example, the origins of life on Earth. According to orthodox biology today, 3.6 billion years ago the first living cell emerged from the dust of the Earth and began to replicate itself, as did its progeny. Eventually, over the course of billions of generations and countless genetic mutations, every living organism—every microbe, plant, animal, and person on Earth—evolved from that single living cell. At some point in this evolutionary process, consciousness emerged from sufficiently complex electrochemical events in a certain multicellular organism so that, in a very primitive way, it became subjectively aware of its environment and its own physical embodiment as something separate from that environment. Advocates of this view insist that there were no nonphysical influences in the origins and evolution of life and consciousness on Earth, and anyone who questions their account is commonly accused of indulging in magical, irrational, religious, or supernatural thinking—all of which runs contrary to scientific inquiry.

Such dogmatism, which is all too often conflated with science, is called scientism: the belief that the natural world consists only of physical phenomena that can be explained according to the laws of physics and biology. Anything else is deemed "supernatural" and rejected out of hand. What advocates of scientism fail to recognize is that the human construct of "the physical" has changed drastically over the past four hundred years of scientific inquiry, and even physicists today do not all agree on its parameters, for, with the advances in twentieth-century physics, many physical entities and processes have dissolved into the realm of mathematical abstractions. This is especially common in quantum physics, where unmeasured quantum systems can be understood only in terms of abstract, immaterial "probability functions," which, when measured, transfer into real physical things. The boundary between "physical" and "nonphysical" has become very nebulous, so it is simply unscientific and naïve to classify as "supernatural" or "magical" anything nonphysical or anything that can't be explained according to the current laws of physics and biology—which are very far from complete! To say that unexplained natural phenomena will all be accounted for according to *future* laws of physics and biology is only an expression of faith in scientism, which should never be confused with empirically demonstrated scientific fact.

From a scientific perspective, the above theory of the origins of life and consciousness is so widely accepted that it is commonly regarded as a well-established fact. No alternative theory seems even remotely viable. But from a contemplative perspective, this is an extraordinary theory requiring extraordinary evidence. So let us review the empirical evidence in support of this view, as if we were evaluating it for the first time. We begin by posing the question: how do scientists define life? There are different scientific schools of thought about the definition of a living organism, some focusing on the cellular level and others focusing on molecular replication. Here is an operational definition of life: a system that is spatially defined by a boundary of its own making and self-sustaining by regenerating all its components from within, with nutrients being taken in and waste produces being expelled through a semipermeable membrane. This definition is common to all living things, including all plants and animals. Even the most primitive single-celled organism has at least a few hundred genes, which means thousands of components, and all these components are interrelated in extremely complex ways.

We then turn to the crucial question: what were the necessary and sufficient causes for the initial emergence of single-celled organisms on Earth 3.6 billion years ago? Scientists have different hypotheses on this. Some, following the lead of Stanley Miller, believe that life first arose from organic compounds in a prebiotic soup. Such compounds are all relatively stable, chemically, so in order to evolve into a living organism, they must be activated by an external energy source, which is what Miller did when he artificially created amino acids fifty years ago.

Other scientists believe that life emerged on a flat area where mineral surfaces could spark chemical processes leading to living cells, which could happen on the ocean floor near undersea volcanic vents. Still others have proposed that the first living cell to appear on Earth actually arrived on an asteroid from some other planet in a faraway solar system. This would imply that the cell survived a journey through billions of miles of deep space, where the temperature is -3700° Celsius (or 3° Kelvin) and then, as its host asteroid passed through the Earth's atmosphere, survived shock pressures of seven and a half million pounds per square inch and shock heating of more than 1000° C, in addition to the shock of impact on the Earth's surface. Quite a sturdy single-celled organism! Of course, even if this wildly speculative notion is true, it does nothing to explain the origins of life in the universe. It simply passes the buck to some distant planet that no one has identified— hardly a scientific explanation! But some advocates of scientism prefer even this over any theory that includes nonphysical influences, indicating the depth of their unquestioning, metaphysical commitment to their ideology.

No one knows whether any of those hypotheses is correct or presently has any way of testing them, for scientists have not yet identified the necessary and sufficient causes of life. Fifty years of attempting to create living organisms from nonliving chemical compounds in a laboratory have met with no success. This does not mean that scientists will never create life in a laboratory, but the fact remains that there is a massive shift in complexity from amino acids that can be made from primary gases to the first living, replicating form, and all the above theories are just hypotheses, without any empirical validation.

All this in no way shakes the faith of those who are committed to this materialist, mechanistic view of the origins of life. Some researchers are committed to designing, modeling, constructing, debugging, and testing artificial living systems. So far, they have fabricated individual biological building blocks, but they have yet to create an entirely new, synthetic, self-replicating organism "from scratch." Even so, some are now intent on stitching together lab-designed biological components, or "biodevices," using parts of natural cells to construct hybrid organisms. Such biodevices cannot reproduce on their own—they need to hijack a living cell—so the artificial creation of a living organism remains as elusive as ever.[19]

Although researchers in this field are convinced that a living cell is nothing more than a kind of biochemical machine, validation of their assumption will come only when they create a discrete, self-maintaining, self-replicating, stable organic creature. That hasn't happened yet, so the entire mechanistic, materialistic theory of the origins of life on Earth remains an unsubstantiated hypothesis. From a contemplative perspective, this is an extraordinary theory with almost no corroborating empirical evidence to support it.

We turn now to the question of the nature and origins of consciousness. As noted previously, psychologists and cognitive neuroscientists are virtually unanimous in their belief that consciousness is a physical function or emergent property of the brain as it interacts with the rest of the body and the physical and social environment. They are confident that it is only a matter of time before consciousness will be understood in terms of physics, chemistry, and biology. In the meantime, as mentioned earlier, all subjectively experienced mental phenomena, including consciousness itself, are undetectable using all the tools of physics, chemistry, and biology; and when they are observed directly, by means of introspection, they display no physical attributes at all. So, from a contemplative perspective, this extraordinary claim about the physical nature of consciousness appears to be utterly unsupported by all the scientific and personal evidence available.

While it is obviously true that certain brain functions are *necessary* causes for the generation of specific mental states and processes, no one knows whether they are *sufficient* for producing all possible states of consciousness. Buddhists have known for centuries that every mental state during a human lifetime has a bodily correlate and that altering or damaging certain physical processes may change or terminate their correlated mental states. So the many recent neuroscientific discoveries based on brain scans showing the correlations between brain and mind states simply reaffirm in sophisticated detail what Buddhists have long assumed to be true in principle. Moreover, it has been obvious for centuries that damage to the brain can impair or eliminate specific mental processes, such as vision, memory, and so on, and that intoxicants and hallucinogenic substances can radically alter one's state of consciousness. But Buddhist and other contemplative traditions have experientially explored subtler states of consciousness that are normally accessed only through years of rigorous meditative training and are not dependent on brain function. And they have discovered that ordinary states of consciousness actually emerge not from the brain but from such subtle, nonphysical continua of consciousness that do not cease at death.

Since scientists have no objective means for detecting such subtle states or any kind of nonphysical influences that may contribute to the emergence of consciousness, they commonly discount these possibilities. This is a case of allowing the limitations of methods of inquiry to predetermine the conclusions drawn about the phenomena one is trying to understand. The only way to directly observe phenomena that may indeed be nonphysical—such as mental images, thoughts, and different modes of consciousness—is by rigorously observing one's own mind. But in the 130 years of modern psychology, no one has yet developed any such sophisticated methods of first-person inquiry.

This is not to say that psychologists have not taken other people's first-person reports seriously. For decades they have listened in psychoanalytic sessions, conducted polls, and developed the methods of psychophysics, and on the basis of such reports measured others' attitudes, beliefs, attributions, emotions, pains, and so on. But they have failed to develop any rigorous means of directly observing mental phenomena themselves. Imagine the current state of astronomy if Galileo and all his successors had conducted all their research by interrogating and observing the brain states and behavior of untrained people who occasionally looked up into the night sky and reported to the "scientists" what they observed, while the astronomers cloistered themselves in windowless laboratories!

Since consciousness is invisible to all objective, physical means of observation, it is no wonder that scientists have been unable to define it in the language of the natural sciences. Nevertheless, we are all aware of being conscious of our physical environment and our own bodies by means of our five physical senses, and—to varying extents—we are also introspectively aware of our own mental states and processes. But the defining characteristics of consciousness as we experience them can be expressed only in the language of first-person experience, not the objective terminology of biology.

Over the last 3.6 billion years of biological evolution on Earth, when did the first conscious organisms arise? Since scientists do not know the necessary and sufficient causes of consciousness in any living organism—and cannot objectively detect consciousness even when it is known to be present— they have no way of answering that question. So they simply assume that some early organism with a simple nervous system, such as a hydra, mysteriously became conscious. Likewise, scientists have no idea what the necessary circumstances are for the emergence of consciousness in a developing human fetus, so they don't know when this occurs, let alone when that consciousness becomes uniquely human. Even though ignorance in this regard is almost total, most scientists still cling to the "illusion of knowledge" that whatever the necessary and sufficient causes of consciousness are will turn out to be purely physical in nature. Nonphysical hypotheses are unacceptable, even though the border between "physical" and "nonphysical" remains vague at best.

Many mind scientists believe that understanding consciousness is by far the most challenging task confronting science, but from the early twentieth century until recently, the scientific community has ignored it. Then in 1976, Francis Crick, the codiscoverer with James D. Watson of the double-helical structure of DNA, decided to view consciousness as a biological phenomenon, and this made it possible for consciousness to be regarded as a legitimate object of scientific inquiry. However, despite almost thirty years of continuous effort to understand consciousness within the framework of mechanistic materialism, Crick made virtually no progress.

Some researchers in this field believe that if they can discover a biological explanation for the unity of consciousness—the neural correlates responsible for the coherence of our individual awareness of ourselves and our surroundings—they will be able to manipulate them experimentally to solve the hard problem—the mystery of how neural activity gives rise to subjective experience. But others have argued that the neural correlates of the unity of consciousness are likely to be widely distributed throughout the cortex and thalamus, so it is unlikely that researchers will be able to pinpoint them in a simple set of correlates.

Some scientists and philosophers propose a limited definition of consciousness in people as an awareness of self, or an awareness of being aware. According to this definition, consciousness refers to our ability not simply to be aware of our subjective states but also to attend to and reflect upon those experiences, and to do so in the context of our immediate lives and our life in history.[20] This introspective faculty of awareness has long been thought unique to human beings. But recent research has indicated that not only other nonhuman primates but even rats are able to be aware of and reflect on their own mental processes.[21]

For decades, researchers in artificial intelligence discounted the possibility of such introspection, for it seemed resistant to any explanation within the context of mechanistic materialism. But now computer systems have been developed that can reason about what went wrong in a calculation and consider whether to continue on their current path to a solution or switch to a new strategy. When people do this, we call it conscious, internal awareness introspection or metacognition. When computers unconsciously mimic behavior associated with conscious metacognition in humans, some researchers in artificial intelligence naïvely leap to the conclusion that they have invented introspective machines. Michael Cox of BBN Technologies confidently declares, "I don't think there is an inherent barrier to self-understanding on the part of machines. There is nothing magical, mystical, spiritual or uniquely human about introspection and metacognition." But recall the earlier cautionary note by another expert in this field: "Whatever there is in human–robot interaction is there because the human puts it there."[22] Likewise, the only way a computer could become consciously self-aware would be if its designer programmed it for conscious awareness. But since scientists do not know the necessary and sufficient causes of consciousness in any living organism, they are in no position to create those causes in a machine. If they believe that their machines experience conscious self-understanding, it is they who guilty of magical, mystical thinking, without a shred of evidence to support their belief.

Scientists widely agree that they do not know how the firing of specific neurons leads to the subjective component of conscious perception, even in the simplest case, such as physical pain. There are currently no empirical means that shed light on this problem, nor is there any adequate theory of how an objective phenomenon, such as electrical signals in the brain, can cause subjective experience. Some believe that breakthroughs in this field will come only with major innovations in methods of inquiry that enable scientists to identify and analyze the elements of subjective experience and their relation to the brain. But this will require scientists to closely observe the widest possible range of subjective experiences, which can be done only introspectively. This may require a complete transformation of scientific thought, with repercussions not only for the mind sciences but for biology and physics as well.

A boldness of imagination and intrepid courage are required to challenge the orthodox methods and views of contemporary science. But such trailblazers may take heart from the counsel of the Nobel Prize-winning physicist Richard Feynman:

> It is only through refined measurements and careful experimentation that we can have a wider vision. And then we see unexpected things: we see things that are far from what we would guess—far from what we could have imagined. . . . If science is to progress, what we need is the ability to experiment, honesty in reporting results—the results must be reported without somebody saying what they would like the results to have been. . . . One of the ways of stopping science would be only to do experiments in the region where you know the law. But experimenters search most diligently, and with the greatest effort, in exactly those places where it seems most likely that we can prove our theories wrong. In other words we are trying to prove ourselves wrong as quickly as possible, because only in that way can we find progress.[23]

17

[PRACTICE]

THE EMPTINESS OF MIND

Rest your body, speech, and mind in their natural state, as in the preceding sessions; then steadily rest your awareness unwaveringly, clearly, without any conceptual elaborations, in the space in front of you. When your awareness settles and your mind becomes calm, examine that which has become stable. Gently release your awareness and relax, then once again observe your consciousness in the present moment. Ask yourself: what is the nature of that mind? Let your mind steadily observe itself. Is this mind something that is luminous and still, or when seeking to observe it, do you find nothing?

Closely inspect the nature of your mind that you have now brought into focus. Are there two entities here—you, who have settled your mind, and your mind that has stabilized— two distinct things? If so, examine the nature of each one to see how they differ. But if there is only one entity here—your mind—identify its characteristics. Is this one thing, "the mind," to be found in any one or more of the mental events arising from moment to moment? Or does it exist independently of each of these mind-moments, overseeing and possibly controlling them? If the mind is not to be found in any of the objects that arise to awareness, probe into the nature of that which is observing the objects and see what qualities it has apart from these appearances.

Does the mind have any spatial dimensions, a center or a periphery? In terms of your own immediate experience, see if it is located anywhere, either inside or outside of your body. What is the nature of the mind as an entity existing in its own right? If you can't identify its own inherent nature, then observe that emptiness. If the mind doesn't exist as an entity in its own right, how could it be meditating right now? Who or what is it that isn't finding the mind? Look right at that, steadily. If you don't discover what it is it like, carefully check to see whether this awareness of not finding is itself the mind. If so, what is it like? What are its intrinsic characteristics? If you conclude that it has no qualities of its own apart from appearances, examine the nature of that which has drawn this conclusion. See how your experience of the mind fits into the categories of existence or nonexistence.

You may discover that when seeking out the nature of the mind, you cannot identify it as either existent or nonexistent. If so, carefully examine that which comes to this conclusion. Is it imbued with a quality of stillness? Is it luminous? Is it empty? Investigate the mind until you achieve decisive insight into its nature.[1]

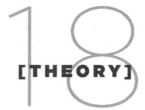

[THEORY]

THE PARTICIPATORY WORLDS OF BUDDHISM

THE SELF-LESS UNIVERSE

At the time of the Buddha, Indian philosophers advocated a wide range of views about the nature of reality. Some claimed that the universe was controlled by supernatural power, either an omnipotent supreme being or a multitude of gods. Some regarded human beings as independent agents who experienced the results of their actions. Some advocated predetermination, declaring that fate, or karma, ruled all things, so humans were deluded to think their choices really made a difference. Others completely rejected any kind of causality, declaring that everything occurred due to mere chance. Despite their differences, proponents of all these views agreed that there was a first cause of the universe, such as a divine creator or an initial, primal substance out of which the world emerged.

The Buddha, in contrast, took the unprecedented view of the universe as a collection of dependently related natural events, not admitting any supernatural influence or intervention by a creator or god existing outside the universe. For example, he attributed the origins of human misery to our own mental afflictions, such as craving, hostility, and delusion, rather than to a God who created the world and punishes us for our sins. All the phenomena within the world could be understood in terms of natural causation, including both mental and physical processes. In making this bold move, he rejected all four prevailing theories of causality.

The way to understand reality as it is, he proposed, was to take as one's starting point the world of experience, rather than an objective, physical world that one imagines to exist independently. On the basis of experience, he sought to understand the reality of suffering, its fundamental causes, the possibility of liberation from suffering, and the path to such liberation. As a result of his investigations, he concluded that the phenomenal world has three fundamental characteristics: all phenomena that arise in dependence upon causes and conditions are subject to change; all experiences tainted by mental afflictions (e.g., craving, hostility, and delusion) are unsatisfying; and an unchanging, unitary, independent self, or ego, is nowhere to be found, not among physical or mental phenomena, or anywhere else. In addition to these "three marks of existence," he spoke of the importance of overcoming the delusion of grasping onto phenomena as substantially existing in and of themselves.[1]

Although Buddhism is widely known for its emphasis on "no-self," this does not mean that the Buddha completely refuted the existence of the self. In fact, on one occasion when he was questioned about the existence of a self, he refused to give either an affirmative or a negative answer.[2] According to his own explanation later on, if he had completely denied the existence of a self, this could have been misunderstood as a form of nihilism or a philosophical rejection of reality altogether—a position he was always careful to avoid.

To understand the meaning of no-self in the Buddha's teachings, consider your own sense of identity in terms of the assumption that you are unchanging, unitary, and independent. Do you think of yourself as having the same, static identity from day to day and from year to year? Are you the same person now that you used to be decades ago? If you think so, carefully examine your body and mind to see if you can find anything that is unchanging. Do you think of yourself as a unified, single self existing separately from the many, ever-changing processes of your body and mind? If so, see if you can experientially identify this single entity called "you." And finally, do you have a sense of yourself as something that exists independently of your body, mind, and environment? Within your own experience, check to see whether there is any evidence for the existence of such an independent ego, either in or apart from your body and mind. For example, can you identify yourself as being identical to any specific function or region of your brain or any other body part? Or are they simply body parts and functions, components of the whole? Likewise, when you observe your thoughts, emotions, memories, and perceptions, are any of them really you? Or are they simply what they appear to be: thoughts, emotions, memories, and perceptions?

Then closely observe how physical and mental events causally influence each other. Examine how one thought influences a later thought or emotion, how your emotions influence your body, and how sensations in your body influence your thoughts, desires, intentions, and emotions. For example, you might have a negative thought about your spouse's behavior, which then puts you in an irritable mood toward your children. This may lead to a buildup of stress in your body, which in turn may cause you to feel judgmental about yourself, resulting in depression and low self-esteem. Can these causal interactions be understood internally—in terms of those psychophysical processes themselves—or do you see evidence that they are controlled or influenced by a separate self or ego that is independent of the body and mind?

In your interactions with other people and the world around you, note whether your sense of yourself as an unchanging, unitary, independent ego acts as a basis for self-centered craving and hostility. For example, when you negatively focus on someone else's faults, do you feel that you are essentially superior to that person, that his faults are intrinsic to his identity, just as your superiority is intrinsic to your true self? Does a sense of your own separate identity raise barriers between you and other people, and does it lock you into the feeling that you can't change, that you are trapped by your own past? All such feelings may be based on a fundamental delusion of mistaking the nature of your own identity. If you identify with your own faults and limitations and think of yourself as the same unchanging person you always were, you may spiral down into a pit of self-condemnation. If you focus on your own virtues while seeking out the faults of others, you will become caught up in a sense of your own superiority, while perpetually looking down on others. Meditation can break up this fossilized sense of one's own and others' identities, showing how we are all in transition—our bodies and minds constantly in a state of flux. We may then be able to stop fixating on others' defects and to freshly and spontaneously re-create ourselves and our relationships from day to day.

The Buddhist view is that no inherently existing self, ego, or soul can be found either within or apart from the body and mind. But this does not mean that you don't exist at all, or that all your thoughts and actions are produced solely by chemical processes in your body. Your thoughts, emotions, desires, and intentions all influence your mental states as well as your body, just as physiological processes influence your mind. You do exist, not as a separate ego, but in dependence upon a collection of mental and physical events, arising from moment to moment and interacting in relation to your ever-changing environment. The more psychologists and neuroscientists investigate the mind and brain, the more they too are drawn to the conclusion that there is no separate self that governs the mind or controls the brain. Rather, mind-brain interactions can be understood internally, with no reference to a self that exists independently of the mind and body.

Buddhism adds the important insight that the innate sense of such an inherently existing self is a fundamental delusion that acts as the basis for craving and attachment to oneself and for hostility and hatred toward others. And these three toxins of the mind—craving, hostility, and delusion—lie at the root of all suffering. When you are hungry, it is natural to seek food, and when you are afraid, it is natural to try to avoid danger. These basic responses are necessary for our survival, and there is nothing wrong with them. The problem comes when we imagine there is an absolute separation between ourselves and others, and then cling to "I" and "mine" with self-centered attachment and respond with hostility and aggression to any "other" who threatens our well-being. Meditation helps us develop a clear awareness of how to take the proper steps to meet our real needs and to avoid danger, without falling into unhealthy attachments that will only cause us suffering.

To take a practical example, while sitting quietly in meditation, recall an occasion when someone offended you, with either their words or their deeds. Think of a time when you were ridiculed or abused, and let your emotions of pain and possibly anger arise. Then carefully examine the sense of self that arises: who is it that is hurt, offended, and angry? Is it your body? Your mind? Or do you have a sense that the person who is responding to such injury is separate from your body and mind? Is this sense of yourself as an independent ego an illusion, or can you find a basis for it in reality? Then take this practice into your daily life, and as soon as you come into a situation where you feel a strong ego response, check out the nature of that strong sense of "I." That sense certainly does exist. But is there really any being that corresponds to the subjective experience of an "I," of your own identity, or is it an illusion? Likewise, when you feel that you are either in control or out of control of your mind, check carefully to see if you really do exist as an independent agent in charge of your body and mind.

The stronger your feeling of being an independent ego, the more likely you are to feel offended by others' rude or mean remarks. It is natural to feel offended and to feel justified in trying to protect yourself. But think of all the time and effort you have given to changing other people's behavior, and then consider how effective you have been. Have you found that rude people really want to follow your advice, especially when you give it to them with a sense of your own moral superiority? In a close and loving relationship, such as a marriage or friendship, there is certainly a place for helping someone else to modify their behavior so that it causes less harm to themselves and others. This is part of true friendship. But most other people don't want our advice, so if we can avoid being offended by their behavior in the first place, we save ourselves a lot of wear and tear. Why should we suffer from other people's misguided attitudes and behavior when we have enough troubles of our own?

Buddhist contemplatives have inquired into the self for centuries, and they have come to the conclusion that no such independent self is ever found. Such experiential inquiry is a direct path to unveiling the illusion of an unchanging, unitary, independent self and liberating oneself from it.[3] The same type of analysis can be used for probing the nature of all other phenomena. For instance, the Buddha pointed out that a chariot, like the self, does not exist as a substantial thing apart from or in addition to its various parts.[4] Nor is the chariot to be found among any of its individual components, and the whole heap of those components by themselves does not constitute a chariot. The term "chariot" is something we use to designate a collection of parts, none of which, either individually or collectively, is a chariot. The chariot comes into existence only when we call those parts a chariot. In the same way, the term "I" is used to designate the body and mind, which are not, by themselves, a real self. "I" come into existence only when I am conceptually designated as such. When we use these concepts and conventions, including the words "I" and "mine," we tend to grasp onto the concepts as being real, independent of our projections. And this leads to endless suffering. Those who are free of delusion still use those concepts and words, but they are not fooled by them.[5]

There is nothing wrong with using these words. Problems arise only when we latch onto "I" and "mine" as being absolutely real and separate from all other beings. This is what creates our sense of an absolute division between ourselves and others, which is the root of racism, ideological intolerance, and conflicts of all kinds. Although all the things we think of and name appear to exist from their own side by their own inherent nature, they are all "empty" of such an essence. They are not absolutely separate from us, so they are not the "real," objective causes of our happiness and pain. Our thoughts and attitudes are entangled with everything we experience. When we realize that, we can begin to lessen our disappointments and frustrations by changing our own minds, rather than waiting for the external world to change according to our wishes.

The appearances of all these objects of the mind are illusory in the sense that they appear to exist by their own nature, independently of our perceptions, thoughts, and language. But in reality, everything we experience arises only in relation to these subjective frames of reference. In that sense, everything we perceive may be regarded as "empty appearances" similar to those in a dream. They seem to be absolutely objective, but they are "empty" of inherent existence in and of themselves. In order to fully awaken to the ultimate nature of phenomena, one must realize the empty nature not only of the self but also of the mind and all the physical elements of the universe.[6]

If all phenomena are empty of an inherent self-nature, how do they exist, how can they function? This is where the Buddha's teachings on dependent origination come in. All impermanent phenomena arise in dependence upon prior causes and conditions. But such causality does not consist of absolutely objective interactions among real phenomena. For example, when the Buddha was asked whether suffering was caused by oneself, by someone else, by both, or by neither, he denied all four of these alternatives. In the ongoing continuum of your personal existence, if you at the time of engaging in a certain act and you at the time of experiencing the consequences of that act are one and the same, this would imply that you exist as an unchanging entity that persists through time. But there is no evidence of such an immutable ego or self. Every element of your body and mind is constantly in a state of flux, with nothing remaining the same from moment to moment. However, if you think that your identity when you perform an action and your identity when you experience its results are totally different, then you are ignoring the unique continuum of your mindstream and the coherent, lawlike causal relations that connect your later experiences to your earlier ones.

There are certainly many factors that contribute to the generation of suffering, such as illness, weapons, natural disasters, other people's behavior, and our own thoughts and deeds. All of these influences *contribute* to the experience of suffering, but suffering itself does not inherently arise from any of those factors. In addition to prior causes—such as illness, natural calamities, and war—its very existence depends on the label of "suffering" that we project onto our experience.

This may more easily be understood in the case of the creation of a chariot. As you gradually assemble the wheels, the chassis, and the seat, exactly when does it become a chariot? When you can roll it? Or when it performs the function of a chariot? In order to know that, you have to know what you mean by the word "chariot." That means that this assemblage of parts actually becomes a chariot only when you project the thought or label "chariot" on those parts. But independently of that subjective designation, the parts do not become a chariot all by themselves. Likewise, if you gradually disassemble a chariot, it ceases to be a chariot only when the designation "chariot" is withdrawn. The existence and nonexistence of a chariot depend not only on its objective causes, parts, and attributes but also on the thoughts "This is a chariot," and "This is no longer a chariot."

The same is true for subjective events such as suffering. Since it, like all other phenomena, has no inherent nature of its own, independent of all labels and concepts, it doesn't absolutely arise from itself, from something else, from both, or from neither. Likewise, when suffering arises, it becomes "my" suffering only when I grasp onto it as "mine." There is nothing in the nature of suffering itself that makes it mine. But when I identify with it as mine, it is experienced as such. A mother may similarly identify with her child's suffering and experience it almost as vividly herself. But she doesn't experience other children's suffering so intimately, for she doesn't regard them as hers and therefore doesn't identify so strongly with their joys and sorrows. The Buddha certainly wasn't refusing to admit the existence of suffering; but he was challenging the assumption that it inherently arises in dependence upon itself or any other inherently existing phenomenon. In another dialogue he similarly rejected the assumption that happiness inherently arises in any of those four ways.[7]

Insofar as we see that our joys and sorrows don't exist inherently, but only in relation to the ways we regard them, we stop being victims of our own feelings and emotions. They don't come to us all by themselves; rather, we experience them in accordance with our attitudes toward them. Insofar as we don't identify with them, but simply observe them arise within our experience, they don't overwhelm us. Then we can learn to deliberately adopt fresh attitudes toward our emotions. We can use our pain to develop greater empathy and compassion for others, and when joy arises, we can offer this to others, rather than trying to cling to it to make it last. At times, there is little we can do to alter our environment or other people's behavior, but we can change our experience of events and our emotional responses to them by shifting our own ways of thinking about them. This is a practical route to freedom. There is a whole genre of practices within Tibetan Buddhism known as "mind training" (*lojong*) that is about changing our experience of happiness and suffering by altering our attitudes about them. Realizing the noninherent nature of our feelings and emotions is central to all these practices.[8]

Nothing exists by its own independent nature, so it can't produce anything else that exists in and of itself. Relatively speaking, things do arise in dependence upon causes and conditions. But they also depend for their existence on their own parts and attributes. A chariot, for instance, is created by a carpenter, but its existence also depends on its parts, such as its chassis, wheels, and seat. Moreover, in order for anything to exist, it must be labeled for what it is. If there were only a chassis, wheels, and seat, it wouldn't be a chariot until someone labeled it as such. Likewise, the body and mind are not inherently a person, but "I" come into existence when this label is imputed upon a body and mind. Even space and time have no absolute existence, independent of the mind that conceives of them. As soon as we label things in accordance with accepted usage, then they can be said to exist within that conventional framework. But, despite illusory appearances to the contrary, nothing exists independent of all such frameworks of language and thought.[9]

A WORLD OF ILLUSION

Although the Buddha's teachings recorded in the Pali language include explanations of the empty, insubstantial nature of all phenomena, not just the lack of inherent identity of persons, many Mahayana discourses attributed to the Buddha elaborate on this theme in much greater detail. These teachings are thought to express the "Perfection of Wisdom," for they shed light on the fundamental nature of reality. The delusion of inherent existence acts as the basis for clinging to ourselves as absolutely separate, independent agents. That, in turn, creates the illusion of an absolute division between ourselves and others. That leads to attachment to "our" side and defensiveness and hostility to the "other" side, resulting in anxiety, frustration, and conflict. And the consequence of this entire sequence of dependently related events is endless suffering. Realizing the profound interdependence of all beings together with our natural environment is the key to freedom from suffering. For this reason it is called the Perfection of Wisdom, the pinnacle of all Buddhist teachings.

One of the most renowned Mahayana discourses is the *Diamond Cutter Sutra,* which has been studied, practiced, and revered throughout Asia for two millennia.[10] Here the Buddha declares that in order to achieve perfect enlightenment one must realize that no object of awareness exists independently of the awareness of it. Perceptual objects, such as sights and sounds, do not exist independently of the faculties by which they are experienced. And conceptual objects, such as electromagnetic fields and gravity, do not exist independently of the minds that conceive of them. For example, when a tree falls in a forest, it makes no sound unless someone has ears to hear it. Animals and humans hear the sound in relation to their own auditory faculties. A fox, for instance, will hear the sound differently from how a snake hears it. When a tree falls in the forest, we modern science-influenced humans say it produces ripples in the atmosphere, or "sound waves," whether or not those ripples strike someone's eardrums. But scientific theories and mental images of wave propagation exist only in relation to the minds that conceive of them. Some intelligent, extraterrestrial beings might visit Earth and conceive of "waves" very differently from the way contemporary scientists conceive of them. Therefore, it is meaningless to speak of waves independently of conceptual frameworks and languages.

All objects of the mind appear to exist independently, from their own side, but this is an illusion. And our subjective minds seem to exist independently from their own side. That too is an illusion. But this doesn't mean that the mind and all objects of the mind are utterly nonexistent. Rather, they exist as appearances to the mind—a mind that also has no existence independent of the appearances to it. This is the ultimate nature of all phenomena, and it is said that one who realizes this "knows the Buddha." This discourse from the *Diamond Cutter Sutra* concludes with the verse:

All conditioned phenomena are like
A dream, an illusion, a drop of dew,
And a flash of lightning.
Contemplate them in this way.[11]

These teachings of the Buddha, first written down in India two thousand years ago, later made an enormous impact on the culture and spiritual heritage of Tibet, where they have been preserved and practiced for over a thousand years. Dudjom Rinpoche, an eminent twentieth-century Tibetan contemplative scholar who was regarded as a reincarnation of Düdjom Lingpa, explained how to establish the nature of objects that appear to our minds as being external:

All animate and inanimate phenomena, including oneself and others, and
things that are designated and characterized as obstacles, demons, and hin-

drances, seem to be truly existent. However, apart from the deceptive appearances of one's own mind there is nothing whatever that exists in reality. Things do indeed appear, but they are not real.[12]

The things we perceive in a dream seem to really exist "there," and we experience ourselves in a dream as really existing "here," wherever we are located in the dream. But all such appearances are illusory. You may walk over to a person in your dream, touch him to see if he's real, and feel the firmness of his body. But there's no real body, existing independently of your awareness of those visual and tactile sensations. Those sensory appearances are "empty" of substantial, absolutely objective existence. And your own physical presence in a dream as really existing is equally illusory. All these objective and subjective appearances exist only in relation to your awareness of them. They are not inherently real, yet you can recognize meaningful, causal relationships among the events that take place in a dream. Likewise, in the waking state, the things we experience objectively and our sense of our own identity appear to exist as realities from their own side. But all such waking appearances are illusory. The primary difference is that appearances in the dream state are products of our own individual awareness alone, whereas appearances in the waking state arise from a deeper, more collective source that will be discussed below in the concluding chapters.

How might we get beyond our erroneous way of experiencing "reality"? Dudjom Rinpoche explains how to establish the nature of the mind, which we take to be internal:

> Without bringing anything to mind, place your awareness in an uncontrived, relaxed state. With your attention directed inward, focus completely on the mind's own nature. By so doing, there will arise a "self-clarity" that is without object, free of the extremes of conceptual elaborations, and free of any sense of apprehender and apprehended, including any viewer and viewed, experiencer and experienced, and subject and object. Freshly enter into meditative equipoise in that very state, without contriving anything, or contaminating or changing it.[13]

These two passages cited from the writings of Dudjom Rinpoche summarize the meditation explained in the previous chapter. They synthesize the very essence of meditation on the Perfection of Wisdom and are designed to cut through the delusion of grasping onto the real, inherent existence of objective and subjective phenomena, which lies at the root of all suffering.

All prior Buddhist practice, including training in ethics, single-pointed attention, and observing the mind, leads up to such meditation. However, it is important to know that although books such as this one may give you some idea of how to engage in meditation, there is no substitute for the personal guidance of an experienced teacher.

In another approach, the nature of all inner and outer phenomena may be realized by closely examining how they initially arise, how they are present once they have arisen, and how they vanish. This careful investigation can be applied both to the objects that appear to the mind and to your mind itself. In this way you may discover for yourself that nothing inherently arises from itself, from something else, from both, or from neither.[14] You do not exist in either external or internal phenomena, nor do external and internal phenomena abide in you. The sense of self and appearances to the self arise spontaneously, but they have no location inside or outside.

The basis of the mind and everything that appears to it is the space of the mind known as the substrate. During the daytime, all the elements of the physical world, all sensory appearances, and all mental events are displayed in the domain of this space and are grasped by the conceptual mind. In the dream state as well, all the events arise from, are then present in, and finally dissolve back into that space of the mind. The nineteenth-century Tibetan master Düdjom Lingpa commented on this point:

> Therefore, space, oneself, others, and all sense objects are of one taste; they are certainly not separate. Moreover, it is the luminosity of space itself, and nothing else, that makes appearances manifest. The essential nature of the mind and its ground is space itself. Various appearances occur in the realm of mental cognition—limpid, clear, forever-present consciousness. The display of those appearances is like the reflections in a mirror or the images of planets and stars in a pool of limpid, clear water. Once limpid, clear consciousness has withdrawn into the central domain of pervasive, empty space, it has been directed inwards. At that time, the mind and all appearances disappear as they infinitely diffuse into an ethically neutral, pervasive void. Through the power of self-grasping, the essential nature of this great, pervasive vacuity, the basis of phenomena, arises as the mind and its thoughts. This is certain.[15]

This passage refers to the space of the substrate, a luminous, empty space from which all objective and subjective appearances arise, as discussed in chapter 12. When we wake up in the morning, all sensory appearances of the world around us arise from and within the space of our own substrate. Like holographic images, sights, sounds, smells, tastes, and tactile sensations do not exist by themselves in the objective world independently of this space of the mind, even though they appear to be totally "out there." Likewise, all our discursive thoughts, mental images, desires, and emotions arise within the substrate. When we fall into deep, dreamless sleep, all sensory and mental appearances dissolve back into the substrate, and when we dream, all dream appearances arise in the substrate like the reflections in a mirror or the images of planets and stars in a pool of limpid, clear water.

The very division between subject and object occurs due to the primary cause of grasping onto ourselves as independent agents. Then the secondary cause—conceptualization—triggers the emergence of appearances from space. When we withdraw our conceptual designation of something as existent, it appears to deteriorate or vanish altogether. All phenomena are mere appearances arising from dependently related events, and nothing more, and nothing whatever is truly existent from its own side.[16]

These themes of emptiness and dependent origination, tracing back to the original teachings of the Buddha, have parallels in the history of European philosophy and science. One of the first was the philosophical movement of empiricism, which began in the fourteenth century with the writings of the Franciscan friar William of Ockham (ca. 1285–1349). This is a philosophical theory of knowledge that emphasizes the role of experience, especially sensory perception, in the formation of ideas, while discounting the notion of innate ideas. Empiricism has been interpreted in various ways by generations of philosophers since the eighteenth century, and advances in twentieth-century physics have invigorated this view, leading to conclusions remarkably similar to those of Buddhism.

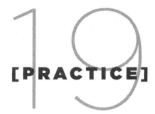

[PRACTICE]

THE EMPTINESS OF MATTER

Rest your body, speech, and mind in their natural state, then place your awareness in repose—unwaveringly, clearly, without any conceptual elaborations, without having anything on which to meditate—in the space in front of you.

Now direct your attention to an object in the physical world, such as your own body. Examine the appearances you designate as "body." Directly, with as little conceptual overlay as possible, observe the visual appearances of the body and the tactile sensations inside and on the surface of your body. Is any of these individual appearances actually your body? Or are they simply appearances, each having its own name? The visual appearance of the arm is just a visual appearance of an arm, not a body. Likewise, the tactile sensations of solidity, warmth, and movement within the body are simply tactile sensations, not a body. If you examine the individual constituents of the body, you will find that each one has its own name, yet none of them is your body. Apart from all those constituent parts and qualities, apart from those individual appearances, can you identify your body as a distinct entity that *has* those attributes and *displays* those appearances? What is the nature of the body as a real thing, existing on its own? Is that anywhere to be found, either among its parts or separate from them? Or, in the process of this investigation, are you finally left with a "not-found," an emptiness of the body, in which not even its label remains?

Consider all the elements of your immediate experience of the physical world: things that are solid, fluid, warm, or cold, and things that are in motion. When you seek out their real, inherent nature, can you find it among their constituent parts or separate from them? Does anything bear its own intrinsic qualities, or are they all simply labels projected upon illusory appearances? Even the category of "appearances" is a human construct. Likewise, the categories of "subject" and "object" and even "existence" and "nonexistence" are creations of the conceptual mind, and they have no existence apart from the mind that conceives them.

Even if you conclude that all these appearances are unsubstantial and empty, consider whether this label of "emptiness" is anything more than a word, a concept. In the formation of the world of experience, we first grasp onto our own self-existence, and on that basis we identify other things as existing apart from ourselves. They are brought into existence by the process of conceptually identifying objects on the basis of mere appearances to awareness. Once we have bracketed an object with our thoughts by labeling, it seems to exist independently of our thought processes. Then, when appearances change and we withdraw our conceptual projection of an object, it seems to vanish. All phenomena are mere appearances arising from dependently related events, and nothing more. Upon careful examination, we find nothing whatever that is truly existent from its own side.

Moreover, when you fall asleep, all objective appearances of waking reality—including the appearances of the inanimate world, the beings who inhabit the world, and all the objects that manifest to the five senses—dissolve into the vacuity of the substrate. Then, when you wake up, the sense of "I am" reasserts itself, and from the appearance of the self, as before, all inner and outer appearances—including those of the inanimate and animate world and sensory objects—emerge like a dream from the substrate. In the midst of these inner and outer appearances, we identify with some as "I" and "mine" and grasp onto others as existing by their own nature. In this way, we perpetuate the delusion of the inherent nature of all phenomena. Only with the recognition of the empty, luminous nature of the mind and all appearances do we find release from that delusion and come to see reality as it is.[1]

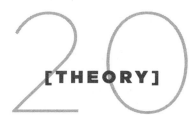

[THEORY]

THE PARTICIPATORY WORLDS OF
PHILOSOPHY AND SCIENCE

A WORLD OF EXPERIENCE

By the early half of the eighteenth century, the many triumphs of classical physics, as formulated by Newton, gave most scientists and philosophers in the West confidence that science was now penetrating to the very nature of the physical world as it exists in itself, independently of all modes of observation and thought. The initial quest of Galileo and other pioneers of the scientific revolution to view the universe from a God's-eye perspective seemed to be paying off. Physicists believed they were now fathoming the nature of the objective world as God himself created it. This philosophical view is known as metaphysical realism, and it asserts that the world consists of mind-independent objects; there is exactly one true and complete description of the way the world is; and truth involves some sort of correspondence between an independently existent world and a description of it.[1] For scientists, this means that the objects of scientific inquiry are describable, in principle, in and of themselves; and they are believed to exist objectively—independently of any descriptions or interpretations imputed upon them by any subjects.[2]

The Irish philosopher George Berkeley (1685–1754) responded to this view with deep skepticism, and he advanced the empiricist concept of knowledge in a radically new way. At the age of thirty-six, Berkeley earned a doctorate in divinity, and thirteen years later he was appointed as a bishop in the Church of Ireland. He wondered: if all of our theories are appearances based on observations and human concepts, how do we know whether they truly *re-present* anything in the real world as it exists apart from our observations and ideas? Berkeley's answer was that there was no way to verify or refute such a correspondence between human theories and the objective world of nature. Physicists assume that all their observations are caused by physical objects, but he proposed that something else might give rise to these phenomena. Berkeley proposed that God was generating appearances of physical objects to our minds without ever creating any physical objects at all, a view known as subjective idealism.[3] According to this view, one's perception of the tree is an idea that God generates in one's mind, and the tree continues to exist in God's omniscient mind when you are not there to witness it. In short, the mind of God directly generates all our experiences of the world, without ever creating an absolutely objective physical world as the basis for sensory perceptions.

In this idealist version of empiricism, the only objects we know and experience are those that we perceive. So everything we refer to as a "real" or "material" object consists of nothing other than these contents of our own perception. Berkeley's philosophy is summed up in the principle *Esse est percipi* ("To be is to be perceived"), which means that we can directly know only our own perceptual sensations and ideas of objects, and not independent, objective entities that we call "matter." Three fundamental assertions provide the framework of his philosophy: any knowledge we have of the world is to be obtained only through direct perception; false ideas about the world are a result of thinking about what we perceive; and our knowledge of the world may be purified and perfected simply by stripping away all thought, and with it language, from our pure perceptions. If we would pursue such pure perceptions, he argued, we would be able to obtain the deepest possible insights into the natural world and the human mind.

This ideal met with a cool reception from both scientists and Western philosophers, though the notion that knowledge of the world may be perfected by purifying our perceptions is common in Buddhism. Among the three primary approaches to knowledge in ancient India—based on people or texts that are regarded as authorities, on logical reasoning, and on direct perception—the Buddha emphasized the development of the third. In particular, he proposed that direct observation of the mind and its relation to sense experience was an especially effective means for acquiring knowledge of reality as it is.[4] The greatest source of error, according to Buddhist tradition, stems from our conceptual projections onto the world, and nirvana is to be achieved by direct, nonconceptual experience.

Immanuel Kant (1724–1804), one of the most brilliant and influential European philosophers of the modern era, rejected Berkeley's subjective idealism, but he too was profoundly skeptical of the notion that we can know anything about the world as it exists independently of our perceptions and ideas. Brought up in a deeply religious Christian household, emphasizing intense devotion and a literal reading of the Bible, Kant eventually became highly critical of the religious norms of his day, though he never abandoned his belief in God. In his philosophy, everything we observe consists of appearances that arise in relation to our methods of observation, and all our concepts of the objective world are likewise bound up with human intelligence and do not represent physical realities as they exist in themselves. Likewise, when we observe our own mental states and processes through introspection, we apprehend only psychological appearances, not an absolutely subjective source of these appearances—namely, a subject that knows, wills, and judges. While Kant didn't deny the inherent existence of things, he did reject the possibility of our ever knowing them either through direct observation or by way of logical inference.[5]

Despite the questions raised against metaphysical realism by such philosophers as Berkeley and Kant, it remained the dominant worldview among scientists through the nineteenth century. But in the early twentieth century, William James developed a new philosophy of radical empiricism, which, as we saw earlier, rejects the absolute duality of mind and matter in favor of a world of experience. In his view, consciousness does not exist *as an entity in and of itself*, nor is it a function of matter, nor does matter exist *as an entity in and of itself*. The very categories of mind and matter are conceptual constructs, whereas pure experience, which is neutral between the two, is primordial.[6] This hypothesis bears a strong similarity to a conclusion drawn by Buddhist contemplatives on the basis of their experiences in deep *samadhi*.[7]

Empiricist critiques of metaphysical realism continue to be presented by contemporary philosophers, such as Bas C. van Fraassen of Princeton University. An adult convert to Roman Catholicism, van Fraassen points out that ever since the fourteenth century, philosophical battles have been waged between empiricists and metaphysical realists. The latter think of philosophy and science as jointly trying to uncover what is really going on in nature, independently of human observations and thinking. Empiricists, in contrast, call us back to experience, while adopting a skeptical attitude toward the philosophical and scientific accounts of why experience must be this way or that. Van Fraassen argues that all science can really do is provide us with intelligible accounts of empirical evidence, without presuming to describe or explain what goes on independently of experience.[8]

Charles M. Taylor is another contemporary philosopher, also a devout Roman Catholic, who takes a critical view of metaphysical realism, especially regarding human identity. Having taught at Oxford University, McGill University, and Northwestern University, in 2007 he was awarded the prestigious Templeton Prize for Progress Toward Research or Discoveries About Spiritual Realities. In his influential work *Sources of the Self: The Making of the Modern Identity*, Taylor presents four attributes that are generally believed to be true of objects of scientific study: the object of study is to be taken "absolutely," that is, not in its meaning for us or any other subject, but as it is on its own ("objectively"); the object is what it is, independent of any descriptions or interpretations offered of it by any subjects; the object can in principle be explicitly described; and the object can in principle be described without reference to its surroundings.[9]

Under the impact of the scientific revolution, the ideal of comprehending the order of the cosmos through contemplation came to be viewed as vain and misguided, as a presumptuous attempt to escape the hard work of detailed discovery.[10] However, Taylor warns that by allowing scientific inquiry to dominate our worldview, "the world loses altogether its spiritual contour, nothing is worth doing, the fear is of a terrifying emptiness, a kind of vertigo, or even a fracturing of our world and body-space."[11]

Regarding human identity, Taylor declares that the ideal of modern science is that of a "disengaged self, capable of objectifying not only the surrounding world but also his own emotions and inclination, fears and compulsions, and achieving thereby a kind of distance and self-possession which allows him to act 'rationally.'"[12] But the danger of objectifying the self in this manner is that we may strip our own sense of identity from its qualitative characteristics, which define ourselves as human agents. And the result is that we damage our sense of personhood, especially when the self is reduced to biological processes in the brain. Our sense of meaning comes in part through putting our experience into words, so "discovering" the nature of ourselves and reality at large depends on, is interwoven with, "inventing" the world we inhabit.

Harvard philosopher Hilary Putnam is another prominent contemporary thinker who has deeply pondered our participatory role in cocreating the universe we inhabit. As a practicing Jew, he regards his own religion as a way—though not the only way—of passing on the experience of a connection with God. However, he adds that one can celebrate Judaism's religious and moral achievements without denying that other faiths and peoples also have religious and moral achievements.[13] Like William James, Putnam connects the idea of philosophy's return to common experience with an interest in religious experience. And he agrees in spirit with Charles Taylor that we limit our knowledge of human nature and the mind by ignoring such subjective causal factors as human desires and beliefs, confining our focus to the objective, unconscious workings of the brain.[14]

Putnam's writings on the philosophy of science bear a striking resemblance to the Buddhist views discussed earlier in this chapter, though it seems that he formulated his philosophy without being influenced by any of the contemplative traditions of Asia. He argues that our words and concepts so deeply influence our experience of what we call "reality" that it is impossible for humans ever to observe or represent the universe as it exists independent of our own conceptual frameworks.[15] However, once we have chosen a language and a conceptual framework by which to make sense of the world, we can discover facts about it that are not simply figments of our imagination or artifacts of our methods of observation. In other words, the methods we choose to observe the world and the ideas we choose to make our observations intelligible to us restrict what we can know about reality, but they do not predetermine the answers to our questions. Stars, for example, are causally independent of our minds—we did not make the stars—but we do observe them by way of our human senses, aided by the instruments of technology, and we conceive of them by way of human ideas. Apart from language and concepts, nothing can be said to be true or false, so our ever-growing knowledge of the universe is produced by our experience of the world, with language users playing a creative role in the formulation of reality *as we know it.*

This implies that our perceptions of the world—including those that we make with the use of scientific instruments—are heavily conditioned by our thoughts and assumptions, so they too are subject to error. This point was made long ago by the Buddha, who commented that mistaken views arise not only from speculative thinking but also from uncritical reliance upon contemplative experience. Even what one regards as "direct experience" is subject to error, for it is commonly structured by one's assumptions and expectations.[16] Putnam points out that there is no absolute demarcation between observing and theorizing. Rather, our observations are structured and filtered by our theories, and our theories are based upon our observations. And the world as we experience and conceive of it is a product of our perceptions and thoughts. In this regard, we are like characters in a novel who are writing our own story. This does not imply that nothing exists prior to, and *in that sense* independently of, human experience, but it does imply that the universe *as we experience it* does not exist independently of our perceptual and conceptual faculties. This theme of the participatory role of the observer in the world of experience has gained powerful support from advances in contemporary physics, to which we now turn.

A WORLD OF INFORMATION

Since the dawn of the modern era, scientists have been seeking to understand the nature of the universe as it would be seen from God's own perspective, that is, from an absolutely objective standpoint. As mentioned previously, all the pioneers of the scientific revolution were devout Christians, and the pursuit of pure objectivity was their strategy for coming to know the mind of the creator by way of his creation.[17] This approach to knowledge persisted through the twentieth century, even as many scientists abandoned all religious beliefs. Albert Einstein expressed the ideal succinctly: "Physics is an attempt to grasp reality as it is thought independently of its being observed."[18] And the majority of scientists, from cosmologists to neuroscientists, assume that the world fundamentally boils down to physical entities and their emergent properties and relationships. Adherence to this view is widely regarded as rational, while deviations from it invite accusations of "magical thinking" and irrationality.

If we are to believe that the universe consists entirely of physical entities and properties, we should have a clear definition of "the physical."[19] If we define this category of phenomena as anything that can be detected using scientific systems of measurement and defined using the language and concepts of physics, then mental states and processes, together with consciousness itself, must be deemed nonphysical, for they do not fulfill either of those criteria. And when mental processes, such as discursive thoughts, mental images, and emotions, are observed introspectively, they exhibit no physical characteristics, such as mass, spatial location, or movement. This is a second indication that they are not physical. Despite all such evidence, one may still believe that the mind and consciousness are physical and that this will one day be demonstrated by advances in the cognitive sciences. But that is a faith-based position, not a scientific one. Moreover, it requires quite a leap of faith to believe that the whole of reality conforms to our current notions of the physical, which are limited by our current technology for measuring what we deem to be physical.

Scientific materialists commonly define the physical as anything that can influence or be influenced by known physical entities and processes. Let us set aside for the moment the obvious circularity of this statement, which fails to define physical entities and processes. This mechanistic view assumes the universal validity of the closure principle, which states that only physical phenomena can exert causal influences on physical phenomena. But this principle must be reconsidered within the context of quantum physics, which undermines its validity as an absolute, invariable law of nature. According to quantum theory, the energy-time uncertainty principle allows for violations of the closure principle, leaving open the possibility that nonphysical processes do influence matter. As physicist Paul C. W. Davies writes, "One expression of the uncertainty principle is that physical quantities are subject to spontaneous, unpredictable fluctuations. Thus energy may surge out of nowhere; the shorter the interval the bigger the energy excursion."[20] Such fluctuations may have played a crucial role in the very formation of the universe as we know it, comprising not only the stuff our world was made of prior to inflation but also space-time itself.[21]

Classical physics tells us that an atom is composed almost entirely of empty space, with the nucleus occupying only a minute fraction of that space. But quantum field theory goes far beyond this simple model. In this theory, which unifies quantum physics with Einstein's special theory of relativity, all configurations of mass and energy are reduced to mathematical abstractions emerging from empty space. All physical processes consist of insubstantial "excitations" of empty space, much as surface waves in a pond are excitations of the pond's water. Although empty space is itself shapeless, it manifests as physical forms, thereby making up what we regard as a "real world."[22] This is a far cry from nineteenth-century notions of matter as consisting of chunky bits of real stuff, moving about in absolute space and time.

There appears to be a profound parallel between the Buddhist view explained in the previous section and contemporary physics. Both propose that all phenomena are illusory appearances arising from space and consisting of manifestations of space. All these appearances are therefore "empty" of any real, substantial existence apart from that space. But most scientists still think of space as something purely objective, independent of the minds of all observers. In contrast, the Buddhist concept of the substrate is of a subjective space in which all appearances arise. We shall explore deeper common ground between scientific and Buddhist concepts of space in the following chapters, but both traditions maintain that all phenomena arise from space, despite the differences in the way they understand space. According to the Buddhist view, all notions of space exist only in relation to the minds that conceive them. This has profound implications for scientists' understanding of the physical world, and it has equally important ramifications for our view of our own place in the natural world, as described in the teachings on the Perfection of Wisdom.

The empirical research of Austrian physicist Anton Zeilinger, who stands at the forefront of research into the foundations of quantum physics, has led him to challenge the assumption that the universe fundamentally consists of physical entities and processes. He points out that in classical physics, the physical properties of a system are regarded as primary, and it is assumed that they exist before they are observed and independently of anyone looking at them. Information based on scientific observation is thought to be secondary, for it is only because physical properties already exist that we can obtain any information about them. In quantum physics this situation is reversed. The information of the system being studied is primary, for it exists independently of any particular observations one makes. The physical properties of that system are regarded as secondary, for they are simply expressions of the information about the system that is created by the act of observation.[23]

Zeilinger insists that it is no longer plausible to make an absolute split between the experimenter and the system under experimental study. At the quantum level, one discovers that the universe is not a machine that goes its inexorable way, as Descartes imagined. Rather, the discoveries that scientists make depend on the questions they put about nature, the experiments they design, and the systems of measurement they create. At all stages in this process, scientists are inescapably involved in bringing about whatever they observe.

Zeilinger sums up this revolutionary orientation to understanding the natural world as follows:

One may be tempted to assume that whenever we ask questions of nature, of the world there outside, there is reality existing independently of what can be said about it. We will now claim that such a position is void of any meaning. It is obvious that any property or feature of reality "out there" can only be based on information we receive. There cannot be any statement whatsoever about the world or about reality that is not based on such information. It therefore follows that the concept of a reality without at least the ability in principle to make statements about it to obtain information about its features is devoid of any possibility of confirmation or proof. This implies that the distinction between information, that is knowledge, and reality is devoid of any meaning.[24]

From the time of Copernicus, scientists have sought to understand the world as it exists from God's own perspective, that is, independent of human observation. This is the assumption underlying all of classical physics, as Einstein declared. But, as Zeilinger declares, quantum physics challenges the validity of this entire pursuit. Everything we observe—as scientists or nonscientists—exists only in relation to our mode of observation, and everything we conceive of exists only in relation to our ways of thinking. We have no observational or conceptual access to any absolutely objective reality, so if we make claims about what exists in the absolutely objective world, we have no way of confirming or refuting them. As Zeilinger maintains, that implies that all such claims are meaningless. Buddhism, psychology, and neuroscience tell us that it makes no sense to speak of appearances existing independently from all modes of observation and measurement. Likewise, Buddhism and quantum physics tell us that it makes just as little sense to speak of theoretical entities, such as elementary particles and probability waves, existing independently of the minds that conceive them.

This revolutionary perspective on the universe as fundamentally consisting of information, rather than material particles and fields, suggests that the assumption that physical entities exist "out there," independent of all modes of observation and all conceptual frameworks, is unfounded. This doesn't mean that the entire universe depends for its existence on human observations and concepts. Even if the human race ceased to exist, that wouldn't mean that the Earth, our solar system, the Milky Way, and all other galaxies would disappear. They would continue to exist as they are perceived and conceived by other conscious beings, including animals and extraterrestrial beings. In this way, multiple worlds arise in relation to multiple species of beings on Earth and presumably elsewhere in this vast universe. But quantum physics states that it is meaningless to talk about the universe as it exists independently of *anyone's* observations or concepts.[25]

Nowadays many physicists are engaging in fascinating speculations about the existence of hidden dimensions of the universe, but their hypotheses are usually limited to realities that conform to the human construct of "physical."[26] In light of the above insights from quantum physics, there seems to be no good reason for limiting further investigations to antiquated or even contemporary notions of physicality. Scientists, with their attention fixed on the external, objective world, have thus far disregarded a dimension of space that can be observed "internally," namely the substrate. Mental processes cannot be located as points in physical space, neither in the brain nor elsewhere. So experience compels us to add at least one more dimension to the usual four of space-time, namely the space of the mind, where all mental events arise and pass. All such mental processes may also be viewed as consisting of information, rather than some inherently existing "mental stuff."

Buddhist contemplatives have found that mental events are just as empty of their own intrinsic nature as are physical events, and even the category of "information" has no inherent existence of its own. All such events—mental, physical, and informational—arise dependently, existing only in relation to the means by which they are observed and conceived. Likewise, all systems of measurement—including all modes of observation—exist relative to what they are measuring or observing; and all theoretical concepts—including those of science and Buddhism—exist relative to the minds that conceive them. In this new vision of reality as a world of information, observers play a key role in forming the universe that they take to be real. We are as responsible for the creation of our world as it is responsible for creating us.

A WORLD OF MEANING

A growing number of physicists are coming to the conclusion that information exists as a nonphysical property of the universe, but they remain divided as to the meaning of "information." Some define it in purely objective terms, with no reference to any observer, while others, including the eminent theoretical physicist John Archibald Wheeler, insist that information must be meaningful to a conscious subject. Any real observation of the physical world, he believed, must entail more than the mindless interaction of a physical process and something we have deemed to be a system of measurement. It is, after all, the mind of the researcher that designs a system of measurement and distinguishes between what is doing the measuring and what is being measured. The act of observation must somehow impart *meaningful information*, implying a transition from the realm of mindless events to the realm of knowledge. An interaction in quantum mechanics, for example, becomes a true measurement only if it means something to somebody.[27]

Wheeler's hypothesis about the nature and significance of information in the universe is very relevant to the mind-brain problem. He argues that it makes no sense to assert that meaning, or semantic information, emerges from mindless atoms or quantum processes, and it is just as implausible that meaning emerges from mindless neurons. As physicist Roger Penrose comments, "one needs a theory of consciousness, in effect, to explain the physics that we actually perceive going on in the world."[28] Likewise, one needs a theory of consciousness to explain the relationships between neural functions and mental processes. But no compelling, experientially based theory of consciousness is likely to be formulated by physicists or neuroscientists studying physical processes alone. Any comprehensive theory of consciousness should primarily be based on rigorous observations of the widest possible range of states of consciousness themselves, and not just on the behavioral or neural correlates of ordinary mental processes.

Most biologists today believe that over the course of millions of years of evolution, consciousness emerged entirely from physical processes as an adaptive trait that helped organisms survive and procreate. If so, then it should be possible to understand consciousness simply by investigating the neural processes from which it emerges. Before leaping to this conclusion, however, it is important to note the sequence through which the natural sciences evolved. First came the innovations of the physical sciences with the discoveries of Copernicus, Kepler, Galileo, and Newton; then came the great biological discoveries of Darwin and Mendel in the fields of evolution and genetics; and finally came the cognitive sciences, beginning with the work of such pioneers as William James, Sigmund Freud, and Carl Jung. The sequence of this evolution of human knowledge is clear—from physics to biology to psychology—and scientists widely believe that the evolution of the cosmos has occurred in exactly that order: from inanimate physical objects to living organisms to conscious subjects. Is this a mere coincidence? Or might it be that our view of the evolution of the universe as a whole is a reflection, or a projection, of the evolution of European scientific inquiry into the natural world during the modern era?

In retrospect, it does not appear inevitable that the first great scientists had to be astronomers or physicists. They could have been biologists or cognitive scientists. Darwin's and Mendel's discoveries did not depend on previous advances in physics, and the most innovative theories of James and Freud did not depend heavily on discoveries in physics or biology. If the pioneers of the scientific revolution had been biologists, is it not conceivable that science today might be based on an organic rather than a mechanical model of the universe? And if they had been psychologists, might scientists today not take a radically different view of the role of consciousness in the natural world?

Such hypothetical speculations cannot be answered, but at least they should encourage us to question the presumed coincidence of the parallel between the evolution of science and the scientific view of the evolution of the universe. It is clear that the specific cognitive processes of living organisms arise in dependence upon their brains and nervous systems, but scientists have yet to discover the necessary and sufficient causes of any kind of consciousness. Nor are they able to detect the presence of consciousness in anything. This implies that if there are dimensions of consciousness in the natural world that influence the course of evolution, scientists have no way of measuring them or even knowing of their existence. Therefore, the belief that consciousness arose solely from physical processes is not validated by scientific evidence. Rather, it is a materialistic assumption, simply a reflection of the limitations of scientific methods of inquiry, which are able to measure only physical processes.

Some contemporary physicists go even further in challenging commonplace assumptions about the history of the universe. Applying the principles of quantum physics to the whole of nature, Stephen Hawking of the University of Cambridge and Thomas Hertog of the European Organization for Nuclear Research (CERN) have proposed that there is no absolutely objective history of the universe as it exists independently of all systems of measurement and conceptual modes of inquiry.[29] Instead, there are many possible histories, among which scientists select one or more based on their specific methods of inquiry. Since the dawn of modern science, physicists have been trying to understand the evolution of the universe "from the bottom up," starting with the initial conditions. Today the beginning of the universe is conceived in terms of the big bang. But Hawking and Hertog challenge this entire approach, declaring that like the surface of a sphere, our universe has no definable starting point, no defined initial state. And if you can't know the initial state of the universe, you can't take a "bottom-up" approach, working forward from the "beginning." The only alternative is to take a top-down approach, starting from current observations and working backward. But how you do this depends entirely on the questions you ask and the methods of inquiry you adopt in the present.

When we apply the principles of quantum physics to the entire universe, as Wheeler and Zeilinger also advocate, the whole of nature exists in a quantum superposition state consisting of an infinite array of possibilities. According to Hawking, every possible version of a single universe exists simultaneously in that quantum superposition. When you choose to make a measurement, you select from this range of possibilities a subset of histories that share the specific features measured. The history of the universe as you conceive of it is derived from that subset of histories. In other words, you choose your past.

According to the leading physicists discussed in this chapter, it is becoming increasingly apparent that an understanding of the nature and role of consciousness in the natural world is imperative to understanding the physical universe. Neither physicists nor biologists nor psychologists know when consciousness originated in the course of evolution, or when it first emerges in the formation of a human fetus. So, just as it is impossible to explain the history of the universe "bottom up" without knowing what the initial conditions were, so is it impossible to explain the origins of consciousness "bottom up," without knowing its necessary and sufficient causes. Following the same logic of Hawking and his colleagues, one should study the origins of consciousness "top down," beginning with the observed nature of consciousness in the present moment. This has been the approach of contemplatives East and West throughout the ages, but it is one that remains unexplored by the scientific community.

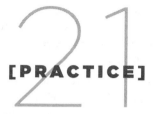

[PRACTICE]

RESTING IN TIMELESS CONSCIOUSNESS

As always, begin your meditation session by settling your body, speech, and mind in their natural states. Once you have gained some experiential insight into the empty nature of objects appearing to your mind, of your mind itself, and of the duality between objective appearances and your subjective awareness, simply rest your awareness without grasping onto any object or subject. This phase of practice is sometimes called "nonmeditation," for you are not meditating on anything. Simply place your awareness in the space in front of you and maintain unwavering mindfulness without taking anything as your meditative object.

In this practice of "not doing," you may simply experience a deep inner stillness. Beyond this, you may break through your psyche and even transcend the substrate consciousness, as your awareness settles in its ultimate ground, known as primordial consciousness (*jñana*). At this time you may nondually realize a steady, luminous emptiness that is the very nature of awareness, beyond all conceptual constructs. Appearances and the mind will merge, so that there is no longer any sense of "inside" and "outside," and you will experience a most profound sense of equality, sometimes called the "one taste" of all of reality.

The luster of this emptiness is unceasing, clear, immaculate, soothing, and luminous. It is called the "luminous nature" of pristine awareness, and its essence is the indivisibility of sheer emptiness, not established as anything, and its unceasing, brilliant, vivid luster.[1] For some people, it may take years of dedicated meditative practice before such a realization occurs. But for others it may arise quite soon. This all depends on our degree of spiritual maturity.

When you bring your meditation session to an end, without grasping, view all appearances as being clear and empty like apparitions or the appearances of a dream. This will help to break down the barriers between your meditative experience and the way you view the world between sessions. In this way, all appearances of thoughts and of the sensory world may arise as aids to meditation. Whatever thoughts arise, direct your full attention to them, and you will find that they vanish without a trace, like wisps of fog vanishing in the warmth of sunlight. Know that these thoughts have no intrinsic reality of their own, and you will no longer be troubled by them. During all your activities, never let your awareness slip back into its previous habit of grasping, but maintain mindfulness, as continuous and unwavering as a broad, rolling river.

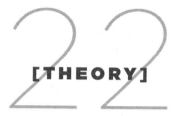

[THEORY] 22

THE LUMINOUS SPACE OF PRISTINE AWARENESS

THE KINGDOM OF HEAVEN

Especially since the rise of the Protestant movement, the Christian Church has tended to characterize human beings as wretched sinners bearing such a corrupt nature that we can gain salvation only due to the undeserved grace of God. While advocates of this dismal view of human nature can certainly find biblical sources for their beliefs, it is important to take into account other scriptural passages that present a more uplifting perspective. The Book of Genesis, for instance, declares, "So God created man in his own image, in the image of God he created him; male and female he created them," and this likeness between God and man is repeated in the New Testament, which states that not only Jesus but all men reflect "the image and glory of God."[1]

Those Christians who emphasize man's depraved nature also advocate their belief that salvation is guaranteed for those who accept Jesus as their savior, receive baptism, and adhere to the beliefs of their church. But such certainty in one's own salvation and in the damnation of everyone who fails to meet those criteria may be called into question when one recalls Jesus' warning, "Not everyone who says to me, 'Lord, Lord,' will enter the kingdom of heaven, but only he who does the will of my Father who is in heaven."[2] Jesus was asked which was the most important of all of God's commandments. "The most important one," answered Jesus, "is this: 'Hear, O Israel, the Lord our God, the Lord is one. Love the Lord your God with all your heart and with all your soul and with all your mind and with all your strength.' The second is this: 'Love your neighbor as yourself.' There is no commandment greater than these."[3] According to Saint Augustine, there is an intimate relation between these two commandments. The love of God is not simply a profound sense of reverence, devotion, and gratitude, but also an ardent desire for union with him. And the love of one's neighbor as oneself is an expression of a sense of unity with all those who are capable of sharing the love of God.[4]

The commitment to seek unity with God with all one's soul, all one's mind, and all one's strength following the will of God accords with Jesus' command, "So be perfect, just as your Father in heaven is perfect."[5] This injunction implies that there is a dimension to human existence that transcends the many limitations and defilements of the human soul. Jesus often referred to this divine purity as the kingdom of God or the kingdom of heaven, declaring that it exists not in the objective world but within each of us.[6] This inner perfection remains obscured as long as we grasp onto our normal sense of personal identity, or psyche, together with all our worldly thoughts and aspirations. To discover the kingdom of God, we must give up our ordinary sense of our own identity, relinquishing our identification with our bodies and minds, for only in this way can we be "born again" and see our deepest nature.[7]

Saint Paul expressed his own spiritual rebirth in his declaration, "I have been crucified with Christ and yet I am alive: yet it is no longer I, but Christ living in me."[8] While Paul remained separate from Christ in terms of his bodily existence, in terms of his awareness, all such separation had vanished. When he looked within, he did not see Christ as an object of awareness. He was speaking of something more direct and immediate, which pertained to the ultimate ground of his awareness. This unifying ground of all unities and communities, the ground of all, is realized only when one breaks through the ordinary mind.[9] Christian theologian Martin Laird comments in this regard, "We realize that what beholds this vast and flowing whole is also the whole. We see that these thoughts and feelings that have plagued us, clouded our vision, seduced us, entertained us, have no substance. They too are a manifestation of the vastness in which they appear. I think St. Paul would simply have called this the peace of Christ, a realization of the baptismal fact of being in Christ."[10]

Many of Jesus' references to the kingdom of heaven were given in the form of parables. He likened it to a mustard seed that is planted in a field.

Although it is the smallest of seeds, when it grows, it turns into the largest of garden plants and becomes a tree, so that the birds of the air come and perch in its branches. Using a similar metaphor of growth, he likened the kingdom of heaven to yeast mixed into a large amount of flour until it is worked all through the dough.[11] These parables imply that the inner perfection of that kingdom is already present in a subtle way even when we grasp onto our thoughts and ordinary sense of identity. But as we gradually let go of our habitual sense of self and devote ourselves to seeking our deeper nature, it gradually saturates our entire being and reveals itself as our inner refuge. In this way, the kingdom of heaven is like a treasure hidden within the field of one's habitual sense of personal identity. Once it has been discovered, the seeker of truth is happy to give up that field in exchange for the priceless treasure, just as one who discovers a pearl of great value is willing to sell everything they own to acquire it.[12]

Numerous passages in the New Testament also refer to Christ as the light of the world and the light of life.[13] Over the past two millennia, the metaphor of light is perhaps the most commonly used by Christian contemplatives to characterize their deepest spiritual realizations. Although the inner light of the kingdom of heaven is invisible to the ordinary discursive mind, it manifests with increasing clarity to those who cultivate a life of virtue and awaken their contemplative faculties. Saint Gregory of Nyssa called it a "luminous darkness," Saint Diadochos referred to it as "the light of the mind," and Saint John of the Cross said of God, "You are the divine light of my intellect by which I can look at You."[14] According to Evagrius, a Desert Father and follower of Origen, mentioned above, the discovery of this luminous dimension of awareness brings an extraordinary quality of tranquility that persists even in the midst of the mundane activities of daily life.[15]

Saint Gregory Palamas eloquently describes such contemplative realization:

> It is, indeed, incomprehensible how deification can raise the person deified outside or beyond himself if it is encompassed within the bounds of nature. . . . Through grace God in His entirety penetrates the saints in their entirety, and the saints in their entirety penetrate God entirely, exchanging the whole of Him for themselves, and acquiring Him alone as the reward of their ascent towards Him; for He embraces them as the soul embraces the body, enabling them to be in Him as His own members . . . the intellect, because of its freedom from worldly cares, is able to act with its full vigor and becomes capable of perceiving the ineffable goodness of God. Then accord-

ing to the measure of its own progress it communicates its joy to the body, too, and this joy which then fills both soul and body is a true recalling of incorruptible life.[16]

The Christian contemplative tradition went into a steep decline with the rise of the Protestant Reformation and the scientific revolution. One of its last great advocates during the Italian Renaissance was Nicholas of Cusa (1401–64). Nicholas was born and educated during his youth in Germany, but he pursued higher education in Italy, receiving his doctorate in canon law from the University of Padua in 1423. Beginning in 1437, he repeatedly served as papal legate for Pope Eugene IV with the Eastern Church based in Constantinople, and he did so with such skill that the pope nominated him cardinal.

Rejecting the scholasticism of the medieval era, Nicholas made major contributions in the fields of law, theology, philosophy, mathematics, astronomy, and mysticism, earning him a reputation as one of the greatest geniuses and polymaths of the fifteenth century. He contributed to the field of mathematics by developing the concepts of the infinitesimal and of relative motion, and his writings were essential for Leibniz's and Newton's discovery of calculus as well as Cantor's later work on infinity. Long before Copernicus, he asserted that the nearly spherical Earth is not the center of the universe, that it revolves on its axis about the Sun, and that the stars are other worlds. He also maintained that celestial bodies are not strictly spherical, nor are their orbits circular. The difference between theory and appearance, he said, is explained by relative motion. Copernicus and Galileo were aware of his writings, as was Kepler, who called him "divinely inspired" in the first paragraph of his first published work.

While returning from one of his missions to Constantinople, where he attempted to prevent the coming Holy Wars, Nicholas had a mystical experience that led to his writing extensively on philosophy and the contemplative life, deeply inspired by the writings of Saint Augustine and later Neoplatonists. He viewed human knowledge as a collective and unifying activity consisting of three stages. The first and most primitive is the knowledge we gain through our physical senses. Sensory knowledge, he believed, integrates the many appearances that arise to our five physical senses into a unified representation of the world around us. The second is reason, the faculty with which we generate abstract, universal ideas. Such knowledge is enmeshed in conceptual frameworks involving such dualities as "one" and "many," and "existence" and "nonexistence." As such, it gives us an inadequate knowledge of reality, without ever arriving at perfect unity. The third and ultimate stage of knowing entails a kind of understanding that transcends reason and logic. This is a kind of mystical intuition by which we may see through all differences and multiplicity that are conceived by the rational mind. It is only with this faculty that we can come to know God as perfect unity, in which all differences are reconciled in the infinite life, in which all opposites converge, or "coincide."

In order to experientially realize this divine unity, the "face of God," he wrote, "it is for me to enter into the cloud and to admit the coincidence of opposites, above all capacity of reason, and to seek there the truth where impossibility confronts me. And above reason, above even every highest intellectual ascent when I will have attained to that which is unknown to every intellect and which every intellect judges to be the most removed from truth, there are you, my God, who are absolute necessity."[17] Whoever sees the face of God sees all things openly, with nothing remaining hidden. Such knowledge is achieved with divine, "absolute sight," without which there can be no human, "contracted sight." This contemplative God's-eye view of reality is enabled by a kind of sight that embraces in itself all modes of seeing. "In God's light is all our knowledge, so that it is not we ourselves who know, but rather it is God who knows in us."[18] The gate of the "wall of paradise," which closes us off from the kingdom of God within, he declared, is "guarded by the highest spirit of reason, and unless it is overpowered, the way in will not lie open."[19]

Like many contemplatives before him, Nicholas of Cusa presented a path of seeking God within oneself: the path of the removal of limits. In the course of this inner exploration, "you find nothing in yourself like God, but rather you affirm that God is above all these as the cause, beginning, and light of life of your intellective soul. . . . You will rejoice to have found God beyond all your interiority as the source of the good, from which everything that you have flows out to you. You turn yourself to God by entering each day more deeply within yourself and forsaking everything that lies outside in order that you be found on that path on which God is met so that after this you can apprehend God in truth."[20]

Nicholas also suggested that such divine vision can be acquired by directing one's absolute sight to the outer world as a "wonderful path for seeking and finding God."[21] This could be achieved by investigating the nature and conditions of the elements, such as fire, and other material objects, such as wood, stones, and seeds. As the Pythagoreans declared, by so doing, one would find in each of them geometrical forms and thereby reduce them to the fundamental potencies that bring them forth. Had the pioneers of the scientific revolution included this pursuit of knowledge in addition to their rational approach based on sensory observations, the entire evolution of the natural sciences might have taken a far more balanced course, integrating both subjective and objective modes of inquiry. Although many of his mathematical and astronomical insights have been quietly absorbed into modern science, Nicholas's threefold approach to knowledge has been rejected by modern scholars and his contemplative writings have been largely ignored. While modern Christianity has for the most part turned away from that path of contemplative inquiry, there are many remarkable parallels between his insights and those of Buddhist contemplatives, to which we now turn.

BRIGHTLY SHINING MIND

Although the Buddha's teachings strongly emphasize the reality of suffering, with a meticulous analysis of the mental afflictions, such as craving, hostility, and delusion, that are its fundamental causes, there are also many references to what he called the "brightly shining mind." This is a dimension of consciousness that is uniquely pliable and supple, once developed. In the ordinary mind it is contaminated by mental afflictions, but these are not intrinsic to its nature. Rather, they are regarded as temporary, or "adventitious," obscurations, and when those veils of afflictions are removed, this luminous awareness manifests in its full glory.[22]

The Buddha further implied that loving-kindness is a quality of the brightly shining mind, and that this dimension of awareness inspires us to develop our minds and seek liberation. He compared mental defilements to impurities in gold ore, implying that just as gold does not manifest its intrinsic radiance when mixed with impurities, so the intrinsic radiance of the mind is not apparent when it is veiled by afflictions. The process of meditative development is therefore likened to refining gold.[23] The discovery of this luminous nature of the mind is crucial to unveiling the hidden resources of one's own consciousness on the Buddhist path, much as the discovery of the kingdom of heaven within is central to Christian contemplation.

Theravada Buddhist commentators identify this brightly shining mind with the *bhavanga,* or ground of becoming, discussed in chapter 12, which naturally manifests in dreamless sleep and at death.[24] During the waking state, ordinary consciousness illuminates all appearances, sensory and mental, but can be dimmed or snuffed out due to damage to the physical senses or the brain. However, the innate luminosity of the bhavanga remains, whether or not it is obscured by mental or physical influences.[25]

This is certainly a reasonable interpretation, but beyond this, the Buddha spoke of an ultimate state of awareness experienced by those who realize nirvana, which he called "consciousness without characteristics," for it is undetectable by all ordinary modes of perception. It can be nondually known only by itself. It persists even after an *arhat* (one who has achieved nirvana) has died, and this unconditioned, timeless dimension of consciousness is imbued with unchanging bliss. In this inconceivable, endless, radiant state of awareness, one is completely freed from physical embodiment: the ordinary mind and body have been transcended and vanish, leaving no traces.[26] The Buddha declared that the consciousness of an arhat who has died is "unsupported," for it has no physical basis, but this does not imply that it doesn't exist. Rather, he likened such awareness to a ray of sunlight that never comes in contact with any physical object and therefore does not "alight" anywhere.[27] Such consciousness transcends all dualities, including that of good and evil.[28]

The Buddha implied that the brightly shining mind becomes this nonmanifestive consciousness, and his teachings support the notion of it as the "womb" of the arhats.[29] As mentioned previously, Theravada Buddhists equate this with the ground of becoming, which is so subtle that it passes virtually unnoticed in the life of an ordinary person. But again, like a mustard seed, when it is cultivated and developed, it turns into the largest of garden plants. Or drawing another parallel with the parables of Jesus, this naturally pure ground of becoming may be likened to yeast mixed into a large amount of flour until it is worked all through the dough.

Ultimately, however, since the bhavanga changes from moment to moment, it is difficult to see how it could stop changing and become an unmoving, unconditioned, nonmanifestive consciousness. Moreover, if that consciousness is timeless, or beyond change, then it must already be present before the arhat dies. It couldn't be freshly created at the time of his or her death, for it is unborn. Indeed, it must be already present, though not manifestly so, before one achieves nirvana, which implies that it must be within every sentient being, regardless of how veiled it may be by mental afflictions.

In fact, the Buddha did emphasize the importance of a dimension of existence that is not born, not brought into being, not made, and not conditioned, without which there would be no possibility of liberation from the cycle of rebirth in a world that is born, brought into being, made, and conditioned.[30] While the brightly shining mind may be identified with the bhavanga at a relative level, its ultimate nature is revealed only when one has fully discovered the nonmanifestive consciousness of perfect liberation. It was there all along, like a treasure hidden within the field of the ordinary mind. As soon as it is discovered, one is happy to give up that field—to spiritually perish and be reborn—in exchange for the priceless treasure, just as one who discovers a pearl of great value is willing to sell everything to obtain it. Despite all the important doctrinal differences between Christianity and Buddhism, the resemblances between the kingdom of heaven within and the brightly shining mind are striking.

BUDDHA NATURE

The theme of the brightly shining mind figures prominently in early Buddhism but is discussed much more fully in the Mahayana discourses attributed to the Buddha. There it is referred to as the buddha nature (*buddhadhatu*), or the womb of the *tathagatas* (*tathagata-garbha*). The term *tathagata*, meaning "one who has reached ultimate reality," is a synonym for a buddha, literally, an "awakened one." In ordinary beings, the buddha nature manifests as we experience ourselves, undergoing the cycle of birth and death, with our minds heavily veiled by mental afflictions such as craving, hostility, and delusion. It is this dimension of our existence that leads to disillusionment with mundane existence and arouses us to seek perfect enlightenment not only for our own sake but also for the welfare of all beings. This aspiration is known as the spirit of awakening (*bodhichitta*), the primary motivation of a bodhisattva, or one who is committed to realizing this lofty ideal. At this point in our spiritual evolution, the brightly shining mind or buddha nature manifests as this spirit of awakening, which reveals its true nature as loving-kindness and compassion.[31] When the buddha nature is fully purified of all afflictions and obscurations, it manifests as the omniscient mind of perfect enlightenment, or the mind of a buddha.[32]

A bodhisattva cultivates a heart of loving-kindness and compassion for all sentient beings, loving each one as himself. So in the Buddhist view, one's "neighbors," whom one is to love as oneself, include not just all of humanity but all sentient beings, that is, all beings who wish for pleasure and freedom from pain. The bodhisattva strives with all his heart, with all his soul, and with all his mind to realize the perfect enlightenment of a buddha, for only by achieving the perfection of wisdom and compassion can one serve the needs of all beings most effectively, leading them on the path to freedom from suffering and to spiritual awakening. So the yearning for perfection is not simply to fulfill one's own aspirations, but to serve the deepest yearnings of all beings. In the often-quoted words of Shantideva, a seventh-century Indian bodhisattva, "For as long as space remains, for as long as sentient beings remain, so long may I remain for the alleviation of the suffering of the world."[33] In the eyes of many modern-day Buddhists, Jesus as the Living Christ is an outstanding example of such an enlightened being who continues to manifest in the world to lead all beings to spiritual salvation and awakening.[34]

The buddha nature is beginningless and endless, and it is blissful, unchanging, and the true identity of every sentient being. Although it is intrinsically pure, it is obscured by mental afflictions, leading us to mistake our own nature as we identify with our faults and limitations. This brightly shining mind is especially veiled by five obscurations: sensual lust and desire, malice, laxity and dullness, agitation, and doubt.[35] This is the same list of five hindrances to achieving the first meditative stabilization given in chapter 10. But here, note that they also obscure the brightly shining mind that inspires us to seek nirvana and enlightenment.[36]

The opening verse of the *Dhammapada*, one of the most renowned among early Buddhist scriptures, declares, "All phenomena are preceded by the mind, issue forth from the mind, and consist of the mind."[37] According to the Mahayana tradition, the mind that precedes all phenomena is the buddha nature, for everything emerges from this intrinsically pure awareness, which is the essential nature of all that exists.[38] This is the one nature of all sentient beings and of the whole universe, and it is indivisible from the absolute space of phenomena (*dharmadhatu*), out of which the relative dualities of space and time, mass and energy, and mind and matter emerge.

Since it is the ultimate ground of reality, the buddha nature holds within it the cause for both good and evil, and like an actor it takes on a variety of forms.[39] It is permanent, stable, and changeless, so it is beyond birth and death. However, we ordinary beings fail to recognize this dimension of our own awareness, so we cling to the appearances of birth and death as we identify with our transient bodies and minds. But our true nature is not different from the omniscient consciousness of the Buddha, forever free of all afflictions and obscurations and imbued with the perfection of all virtues. Although this brightly shining mind is pure by nature, it must be separated from the impurities of mental afflictions, just as gold ore has to be refined to reveal the purity of gold.[40]

Ultimately, the buddha nature, indivisible from the absolute space of phenomena, transcends all dualities, including that of good and evil. The relative

Buddhist teachings on impermanence, suffering, and no-self can be realized with direct perception by carefully attending to the arising and passing of mental and physical events. The ultimate teachings on the empty nature of all phenomena can first be understood using reasoning, which then leads to direct, perceptual insight. The transcendent teachings on the buddha nature can be initially fathomed only with faith, which through diligent practice eventually matures into direct, nondual realization.[41] Such discourses of the Buddha speak directly to our innermost nature, and it is from the intuitive depths of our own brightly shining mind that we may embrace such teachings, even without empirical evidence or logical arguments to support them. These words are spoken from the Buddha's mind to our own buddha nature, which is indistinguishable from the Buddha's mind, so they are expressions of our true self, calling out to itself.

THE GREAT PERFECTION

The Mahayana teachings on emptiness and the buddha nature were thoroughly integrated in the Great Perfection tradition of Buddhism, which is regarded by many Tibetan Buddhists as the pinnacle of Buddhist theory and practice. According to Buddhist records, Prahevajra, the Buddhist contemplative who first taught the Great Perfection, was born as a divine incarnation by way of an immaculate conception to a woman of royal lineage in a region thirteen months' journey to the west of Bodh Gaya (where the Buddha achieved enlightenment). Swiftly recognized as a spiritual prodigy, when he was a child of seven, he was invited to meet with five hundred religious scholars in the king's court. Although the scholars were deeply skeptical, after they had questioned him at length about a wide range of spiritual matters, they held him in awe for his profound insight.

As he grew into adulthood, Prahevajra remained in *samadhi* for thirty-two years, during which neither the blowing of a trumpet in his ear nor being poked with a cane could arouse him from his meditation. When he emerged from this period of solitary contemplation, he revealed the teachings of the Great Perfection. At the end of an exceptionally long life, he gave his last teachings, called *The Three Statements That Strike the Vital Point*,[42] to a close disciple named Mañjushrimitra. He then departed from this world, according to Buddhist accounts, with his body dissolving into an orb of light.[43] There are a number of remarkable parallels between the account of his life and the life of Jesus, and in fact Jesus and Prahevajra lived during the same era.

The practice of the Great Perfection is based on the realization that everything in the universe, including nirvana itself, is empty of inherent nature. Although everything appears to exist by its own nature, in reality all appearances have no existence apart from the buddha nature, which is indivisible from the absolute space of phenomena. All phenomena are like the reflections of the planets and stars in water or like rainbows in the sky. Just as such reflections have no existence apart from the water and rainbows have no existence apart from the sky, so are all phenomena manifestations of the absolute space of phenomena, which is primordially pure and equally present in all aspects of reality.

In the Great Perfection the buddha nature is known as primordial consciousness, which is "the natural glow" of the absolute space of phenomena, manifesting in the aspect of limpidity and clarity, like the dawn breaking and the sun rising. Düdjom Lingpa explains this ultimate dimension of consciousness as follows:

> It is not blank, like an unceasing darkness that knows nothing. All appearances are naturally present, without arising or ceasing. Just as heat is naturally present in the nature of fire, moisture is present in the nature of water, and coolness is present in the nature of the wind, due to the unceasing power in the nature of primordial consciousness, there is total knowledge and total awareness of all phenomena, without its ever merging with or entering into objects. Primordial consciousness is self-originating, naturally clear, free of outer and inner obscuration; it is the all-pervasive, radiant, clear infinity of space, free of contamination.[44]

To realize primordial consciousness, which is the mind of the Buddha, is to realize one's own nature, one's own "brightly shining mind," known in this tradition as "clear light awareness." Such pristine awareness never becomes good or bad, for it transcends all dualities, all conceptual constructs, as the immutable, primordially pure, all-pervasive, absolute space of the whole of reality. This ultimate ground transcends time as we know it, for it is associated with "the fourth time," a dimension that transcends the past, present, and future.[45] There are three indivisible facets to the Great Perfection: primordial consciousness (*jñana*), the absolute space of phenomena, and the energy of primordial consciousness (*jñana-vayu*). This third facet is the life force that permeates the entire universe, manifesting most explicitly in all living things, including plants, while the awareness of all sentient beings derives from primordial consciousness. All other forms of matter and energy (thermal, electromagnetic, and so on) are derivative of this primordial energy, just as all types of animal and human consciousness are derivative of primordial consciousness. All the relative manifestations of space-time in the universe are expressions of the absolute space of phenomena.

Nicholas of Cusa portrayed God as an absolute unity, transcending all opposites, who became "contracted" into the multiple emanations of the world. In his view, the infinite potential of the divine, which is the essential nature of all things, therefore permeates the entire universe, and nothing exists outside of or other than God. Likewise, according to the Great Perfection tradition, the entire universe consists of manifestations of the absolute space of phenomena, indivisible from primordial consciousness. And just as the reflections of the planets and stars in the ocean do not exist apart from the ocean and rainbows in the sky have no existence apart from the sky, so does nothing exist apart from this ultimate ground. The Dalai Lama comments in this regard:

> Any given state of consciousness is permeated by the clear light of primordial awareness. However solid ice may be, it never loses its true nature, which is water. In the same way, even very obvious concepts are such that their "place," as it were, their final resting place, does not fall outside the expanse of primordial awareness. They arise within the expanse of primordial awareness and that is where they dissolve.[46]

Düdjom Lingpa explains that although the absolute space of phenomena, inseparable from the clear light of primordial awareness, is present in the mind streams of all sentient beings, it becomes tightly constricted, or "frozen," by dualistic grasping. When we, as the observer-participants in our world, grasp onto objects as inherently real and separate from our own awareness, they appear as external, firm, and solid. This, he says, "is like water in its natural, fluid state freezing in a cold wind. It is due to dualistic grasping onto subjects and objects that the ground, which is naturally free, becomes frozen into the appearances of things."[47]

Faint precursors of these three facets of the Great Perfection are found in the earlier experiences of the substrate, the substrate consciousness, and the life force (*jiva*). The substrate is like a relative manifestation of the absolute space of phenomena; the substrate consciousness bears similarities to primordial consciousness and is often mistaken for this infinitely deeper state of awareness. And the life force is a faint reflection of the energy of primordial consciousness. These three relative phenomena manifest distinctly, with the substrate appearing as the object of substrate consciousness and the life force permeating that substrate. But in the experience of the Great Perfection, the absolute space of phenomena, primordial consciousness, and its energy are indistinguishable, transcending all conceptual categories.

A similar and related relativism can be found among levels of realization. From the perspective of an arhat, a yogi who achieves *shamatha* and then complacently rests in the substrate consciousness has fallen to an extreme of quietude. For this person is not actively seeking his own ultimate well-being by completely purifying the mind of all afflictions so that the perfect freedom of nirvana can be realized. Likewise, from a Mahayana perspective, an arhat who complacently rests in nirvana has fallen to an extreme of quietude. For this person is not striving for the well-being of all other sentient beings by striving to completely purify the mind of all its subtle obscurations so that the perfect enlightenment of a Buddha can be realized.

Recall that in early Buddhist literature, the brightly shining mind is characterized as the womb of the arhats, or those who achieve nirvana, and in the Mahayana literature this mind is called the womb of the tathagatas, or buddhas. The source of the realization of nirvana and of perfect enlightenment is the Great Perfection. An arhat realizes nirvana as emptiness, which is commonly equated with the absolute space of phenomena. This ultimate reality is absolutely still, inactive, blissful, and unchanging, and this is how nirvana is characterized in the earliest teachings of the Buddha. The final nirvana of an arhat entails a nondual realization of the nonconceptual, primordial stillness of the absolute space of phenomena. But it seems that such a being has not fully realized the perfect luminosity of omniscient, primordial consciousness or the creative potential of the energy of primordial consciousness. One who achieves the perfect spiritual awakening of a buddha, fully realizes all three aspects of the Great Perfection.

The sequence of meditations in the Great Perfection begins with an initial, partial realization of emptiness, like one's first experience of having a lucid dream, in which you know that nothing that appears to your mind exists by its own nature, independent of your awareness of it. On the basis of this first insight, you continue investigating the nature of all kinds of phenomena until you realize that all are empty of their own self-nature. The culmination of this line of inquiry is the recognition of "the one taste of great emptiness," the awareness that everything naturally arises from the expanse of the absolute space of phenomena and does not exist apart from that ultimate ground. Once you have gained this realization, you thoroughly assimilate this awareness until you are never parted from it, either during meditation or between meditation sessions. At that point it is said that you have gained "the confidence of realization." You have now realized the view of the Great Perfection, and when you are on the cusp of such enlightenment you have transcended all preference for ultimate reality over the phenomenal world. All is seen to be of "one taste," everything imbued with primordial purity and equality.[48]

From the time that you identify this brightly shining mind as the mind of the Buddha, your own consciousness is seen as nothing other than an expression of this primordial consciousness. Previously, it was only due to grasping onto your ordinary sense of yourself that primordial consciousness took on the guise of your personal consciousness, like a pile of stones being mistaken for a man. Düdjom Lingpa explains:

> The transformation of that into primordial consciousness is like recognizing a scarecrow for what it is instead of seeing it as a man. In this way, the correct realization of the mode of being of consciousness transforms it into primordial consciousness. It is not that consciousness must vanish into absolute space and primordial consciousness must arise from somewhere else. Instead, know that it just seems that way because of the functions of self-grasping and identitylessness. Consciousness is what makes the first moment of knowledge emerge in the aspect of the object, just as various images of planets and stars emerge in the ocean. What arises is closely held by conceptual consciousness; it is bound by reification, and one thereby becomes deluded. Knowledge of the reasons for that brings one to primordial consciousness.[49]

Our own minds have never been separate from the primordial consciousness of the Buddha, but it appears that they are separate because we grasp onto our perceptions, thoughts, and emotions as our own. In reality, they are identityless, for there is nothing in the mind that makes it intrinsically "I" or "mine." But when we view appearances with our ordinary consciousness, they appear to be separate from us, arising in the aspect of objects, which we then reify, or grasp onto as being inherently real and independent. In this way we become deluded, and the true nature of our own awareness is obscured. By realizing how such delusion arises, we come to the realization of primordial consciousness.

The Great Perfection describes this ultimate reality with various parables, some of them reminiscent of Jesus' parables about the kingdom of heaven. One who is ignorant of their own buddha nature is like a kingdom with no king, but when one identifies one's own pristine awareness, this is like a poor person without any status or possessions being enthroned as a king and enjoying all the privileges of royalty. One who is ignorant of his own true identity is like a person afflicted with a disease, while right under his bed is a medicine that could completely cure the terrible illness. Such ignorance is also likened to the extreme poverty of someone dying of starvation while all the time sleeping on a pillow filled with gold.[50] According to the Great Perfection, the primary difference between buddhas and unenlightened beings is that the former know who they are, while the latter do not. Correspondingly, the root of suffering is grasping onto that which is not "I" and "mine" as being "I" and "mine," while failing to recognize who we really are.

The culmination of the path of the Great Perfection is the realization of the "rainbow body," in which one's body allegedly dissolves into shimmering, multicolored light at death. If the theory of reincarnation stretches the scientific imagination, the Buddhist assertion of the rainbow body transcends all bounds of credulity for many people in the modern world. If such assertions, allegedly based on numerous eyewitness reports, were true, this would strike at the root of many of the most basic scientific assumptions about the nature of mind and matter. Since the inception of the academic discipline of psychology, scientists have been assuming that the mind is nothing more than a function of the brain, and all its influences on the material world are by way of brain functions. Medieval scholastics demanded ideological authority over the whole of reality, so when Galileo demanded that natural philosophers like himself be granted the authority to make their own discoveries based on empirical observations of objective, physical phenomena, he met with fierce resistance. According to the scholastics, the only kinds of observations that were empirically sound were those that conformed to their all-encompassing theological worldview. If Galileo or anyone else claimed to observe things that were incompatible with scholastic assumptions, those observations were dismissed out of hand.

Likewise, scientific materialists today insist that scientists alone have viable methods of inquiry and authoritative knowledge of the whole of reality; any claims of observing things that are inexplicable from a materialistic point of view are deemed invalid and unworthy of serious consideration. Contemplatives challenge this ideological hegemony of materialism much as Galileo challenged the hegemony of scholasticism, and the resistance to acknowledging alternative methods of inquiry is as stubborn today as it was in the seventeenth century. The following discussion of the rainbow body presents Tibetan Buddhist views on the potential of advanced levels of contemplative practice to transform not only the mind but also the body in ways unimaginable to most contemporary scientists. Whether these Buddhist assertions are true or not is to be determined with experience—by putting the corresponding meditations into practice—and not by an appeal to illusions of knowledge about the nature and limitations of consciousness.

Prahevajra allegedly manifested the rainbow body when he left this world, with his physical form dissolving into an orb of light. The mind of such a being who has achieved perfect enlightenment has already dissolved into primordial consciousness, and at death the material constituents of the body dissolve back into the absolute space of phenomena, while the life force dissolves into the energy of primordial consciousness. In rare cases, this complete transference into absolute ground takes place while one is still alive. The mind of one who has achieved the "great transference rainbow body" extends infinitely into all-pervasive primordial consciousness, like water merging with water or space merging with space. All the atoms of the body vanish into the absolute space of phenomena, but one still retains the appearance of a physical body, which can be seen and touched by others. At this point, there is no body or mind that can die—such enlightened beings simply manifest and withdraw the appearance of their bodies in the service of others, but they are no longer subject to either birth or death.

Padmasambhava and Vimalamitra, two great contemplatives in the eighth century who played major roles in bringing Buddhism to Tibet, are said to have manifested the great transference rainbow body. Later lamas said to have achieved this transformation include Chetsün Senge Wangchuk (eleventh to twelfth centuries), Nyenwen Tingdzin Zangpo, and Chetsün Senge Shora, but such accounts are very rare. More common is the realization of the "great rainbow body," manifested by Prahevajra, in which one's body vanishes at death like a rainbow disappearing into the sky. Even more common, according to Tibetan accounts, is the realization of the "small rainbow body." When this occurs, the clear light awareness of the absolute ground arises, emanating the colors of the rainbow from this absolute space, and the material body of the contemplative decreases in size until it finally vanishes without leaving any trace of the body or mind behind. Alternatively, when the clear light of the ground arises at death, the material bodies of some adepts decrease in size for as long as seven days, finally leaving only the residue of their hair and nails behind.[51]

It is said that thirteen of Düdjom Lingpa's disciples manifested the rainbow body at their deaths, indicating what an extraordinarily effective teacher he must have been. More currently, in June 2000, I had the privilege of serving as the interpreter for Penor Rinpoche, the former head of the Nyingma order of Tibetan Buddhism, and on that occasion he commented that he personally knew of six Tibetan contemplatives during his lifetime who manifested the rainbow body when they died. All of these occurred in Tibet. Over the past decade, I've heard of several Tibetan adepts whose bodies diminished in size to only two or three feet in length when they died, with all the proportions of the body remaining the same. These include the late Panchen Lama, a lama named Geshe Lamrimpa who lived in Drepung monastery in Lhasa, and another lama who lived in Dzamthang monastery in eastern Tibet. A fourth lama who manifested this degree of the rainbow body outside of Tibet was Tulku Urgyen Rinpoche, who lived in Kathmandu, Nepal.[52] In all these cases, eyewitnesses reported that at death, these lamas' bodies shrank down to the size of a small child but retained the proportions and features of an adult.

The Tibetan Buddhist description of the great transference rainbow body is somewhat reminiscent of the New Testament accounts of Jesus' resurrection. Three days following his death, it is written, Mary Magdalene and his mother Mary found his tomb empty, with the stone rolled away. Shortly thereafter he appeared to Mary Magdalene, and she reported this to the remaining apostles, who responded with open disbelief. But later the resurrected Jesus suddenly appeared to his apostles, allowing them to touch his hands and feet and eating with them so that they would know they were not seeing a ghost. Finally, when he had led them out to the vicinity of Bethany, he lifted up his hands, blessed his disciples, and was taken up into heaven.[53]

One Christian with an interest in the possible relationship between Jesus' resurrection and Buddhist accounts of the rainbow body is David Steindl-Rast, a Benedictine monk, who commented, "If we can establish as an anthropological fact that what is described in the resurrection of Jesus has not only happened to others, but is happening today, it would put our view of human potential in a completely different light."[54] Brother David asked his colleague Francis Tiso, an ordained Roman Catholic priest who had studied the Tibetan language and culture, to investigate this matter. Father Tiso learned of a recent account of a Tibetan lama in eastern Tibet named Khenpo Achö, whose body vanished after his death in 1998. He then traveled to the village in Tibet where Khenpo Achö had died and conducted taped interviews with eyewitnesses to his death. He reported, "Everyone mentioned his faithfulness to his vows, his purity of life, and how he often spoke of the importance of cultivating compassion. He had the ability to teach even the roughest and toughest of types how to be a little gentler, a little more mindful. To be in the man's presence changed people."[55]

When Khenpo Achö's breath stopped, one eyewitness reported that his flesh turned pinkish, another said it became brilliant white, and everyone there said it started to shine. His body was then wrapped in a yellow robe, and as the days went by, his companions said that they could see through the robe that his bones and his body were shrinking. After seven days, the yellow cloth in which his body had been wrapped was removed, and his body was found to have vanished entirely. In this way he manifested the "small rainbow body," and his dissolution into the absolute space of phenomena was complete.

While Jesus' resurrection is thought by Christians to be unique, the parallels to Tibetan Buddhist accounts of the manifestation of the rainbow body are startling. We may never know whether the Christian resurrection can be understood in Buddhist terms, but it is possible to put the Buddhist assertions regarding the rainbow body to the test of experience. The Great Perfection tradition of Buddhism sets forth a step-by-step path of purification that culminates in this radical transmutation of the body and mind. This tradition has maintained its vitality since the time of Prahevajra, and its claims about human nature and our relation to the universe present an extraordinary challenge to many religious and scientific assumptions that limit the human imagination today.

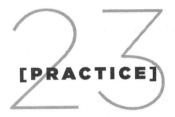

[PRACTICE]

MEDITATION IN ACTION

Between meditation sessions, without grasping, view all appearances as being clear and empty, like apparitions or the appearances of a dream. This will help to break down the barriers between your meditative experience and the way you view the world between sessions. In this way, all appearances of thoughts and of the sensory world may arise as aids to meditation. Whatever thoughts arise, direct your full attention to them, and you will find that they will vanish without a trace, like wisps of fog vanishing in the warmth of sunlight. Know that these thoughts have no intrinsic reality of their own, and you will no longer be troubled by them. During all your activities, never let your awareness slip back into its previous habit of grasping, but maintain mindfulness, as continuous and unwavering as a broad, rolling river.

In terms of your physical conduct, move slowly and serenely, firmly and resolutely. When walking, move deliberately, taking each step in an easygoing manner. When rising, get up slowly, not abruptly, and when eating, chew and swallow mindfully. When conversing with others, speak gently and slowly and avoid pointless chitchat. Adjust your speech so that you express the truth, speaking pleasantly and deliberately, without disturbing the minds of others. Avoid self-praise and pretense motivated by the desire for fame and status. Whatever happens, let your mind be calm, subdued, and spacious, without succumbing to emotional vacillations.

Life is short and precious, so there is no point in pursuing such things as high status, power, or wealth. When you are engaging in meditation, on occasion you may experience an unprecedented, soothing sense of bliss, a pristine sense of clarity, or periods of deep, inner quiet. Do not regard any of these experiences as ultimate realizations, but just let them be without clinging to them, hoping that they will return, or fearing that they will not. Once you have recognized the nature of such meditative experiences, by letting them be in their own state, without attachment, craving, rejection, or affirmation, they will vanish altogether, and the primordial consciousness of awareness will become manifest.[1]

[THEORY] 24

THE UNIVERSE AS A WHOLE

PERFECT SYMMETRY

The scientific revolution of the sixteenth and seventeenth centuries, which began with great breakthroughs in the fields of astronomy and physics, was pioneered by Christians, such as Copernicus, Galileo, and Newton, who believed the universe was created several thousand years ago and would soon end with the Second Coming of Jesus. The universe as they conceived of it, based on a literal reading of the Bible, was created in its present form prior to the creation of humanity. Belief in this account led generations of scientists over the past four centuries to adopt a philosophical stance of metaphysical realism. In this view, an absolutely objective God created an absolutely objective, physical universe, and it was the task of the scientist to try to understand the world from God's own perspective, independent of the limitations of the human mind and senses.

Subsequent advances in astronomy and biology have discredited any literal interpretation of the Genesis story in terms of the age of the universe and the evolution of the human species. The second revolution in the physical sciences that began in the early twentieth century with the development of quantum physics and relativity theory has challenged the assumptions of metaphysical realism. And what of consciousness? In classical physics it is assumed that human consciousness plays no significant role in the formation of the universe as we experience it. Most scientists today believe that human consciousness is simply a natural function or property of the brain. Many Christians, following the lead of Descartes, believe that the human soul is divinely inserted into the fetus at conception. Either way, the emergence of consciousness in the universe is seen as playing an insignificant role in the larger scheme of things.

A growing number of contemporary physicists, however, are beginning to challenge this assumption. Stanford cosmologist Andre Linde, for example, points out:

> The standard assumption is that consciousness, just like space-time before the invention of general relativity, plays a secondary, subservient role, being just a function of matter and a tool for the description of the truly existing material world. But let us remember that our knowledge of the world begins not with matter but with perceptions. . . . We are substituting the reality of our feelings by the successfully working theory of an independently existing material world. And the theory is so successful that we almost never think about its possible limitations.[1]

He then hypothesizes that consciousness, like space-time, might have its own characteristics independent of matter, and that neglecting this will lead to a description of the universe that is fundamentally incomplete and misleading. "Is it possible," he asks, "to introduce a 'space of elements of consciousness,' and investigate a possibility that consciousness may exist by itself, even in the absence of matter, just like gravitational waves, excitations of space, may exist in the absence of protons and electrons?"[2] He hypothesizes that with the further development of science, the study of the universe and the study of consciousness will be found to be inseparably linked, and that ultimate progress in the one will be impossible without progress in the other.

One of the most provocative applications of modern physics to the role of consciousness in the universe is found in the field of quantum cosmology. In 1967, physicists John Wheeler and Bryce DeWitt adapted the primary equation of quantum physics, known as the Schrödinger wave equation, to the entire universe. This unprecedented universalization of quantum theory enables physicists to calculate which events are probable and which are not. One of the remarkable characteristics of this equation is that it does not depend on time, and this implies that an absolutely objective universe, independent of any observer, does not change with time. Physicists call this the problem of frozen time, or simply the time problem.[3] Linde explains, "The universe becomes alive (time-dependent) only when one divides it into two parts: an observer and the rest of the universe. Then the wave function of the rest of the universe depends on the time measured by the observer. In other words, evolution is possible only with respect to the observer. Without an observer, the universe is dead."[4] In his theory of a "self-observing universe," John Wheeler replaces the word "observer" with the word "participant," suggesting that we are inextricably involved in determining the nature of the universe as we experience it.

Following a similar line of thought, Stephen Hawking has argued, as noted in chapter 18, that the observer-participant plays a key role in determining not only the present nature of our universe but also its history as we understand it. Many physicists believe that the universe began in a perfectly symmetrical but unstable vacuum, in which all the forces of nature were undifferentiated. The potential energy of the initial state was like being on top of a hill and the potential energy of the true vacuum was like being at the bottom of the hill. The difference in energy led to the creation of photons, particles, and antiparticles and the reheating of the universe to a very high temperature. As the universe further expanded, it went through several symmetry-breaking phase transitions, which led to the distinction of the energy into gravitational, weak, electromagnetic, and strong forces. The final vacuum we see has much less symmetry than the original, high-temperature vacuum, much as ice is less symmetric than liquid water. As the universe cooled down, transitioning from the state of the "melted vacuum" to the current "frozen vacuum," the initial symmetry was broken in various ways.

According to MIT cosmologist Alan Guth, the theory of an inflationary universe leaves open the possibility that the big bang was not a singular event, but was more like the biological process of cell division. According to this view, the universe is a process that may never have started and will almost certainly never stop. If so, we are dwelling in an eternally self-reproducing universe, with our current universe originating from an earlier one. Likewise, according to Andre Linde, our universe is just one of countless self-reproducing universes, or "bubbles," in each of which the initial conditions differ and diverse kinds of elementary particles interact in different ways. The entire universe may be likened to a cluster of bubbles attached to each other, with each universe emerging from its own big bang involving a fluctuation of the vacuum followed by inflation. This vision of the world we see around us is, as physicist Steven Weinberg has put it, "only an imperfect reflection of a deeper and more beautiful reality."[5]

PERFECT EQUILIBRIUM

In the spirit of Pythagoras, Franklin Merrell-Wolff described his practice as a combination of philosophy, mathematics, and yoga. Although he transcended the duality of subject-object consciousness during his first realization, described in chapter 10, for a period of approximately thirty-three days he remained caught up in an unresolved tension that prevented him from experiencing a yet higher state of consciousness. This tension existed in the contrast between two states of consciousness. The first was his experience of the transcendent, which brought with it a sublime sense of joy, peace, rest, freedom, and knowledge. The second was his awareness of the emptiness of the ordinary world. He vividly experienced the difference between being freed from physical embodiment and having his consciousness bound to a body, and he was subtly drawn to such freedom. However, he overcame this attachment to disembodiment with his acceptance of the bodhisattva vow as it is expressed in Mahayana Buddhism: the commitment to compassionately take physical rebirth in the world—even after one has achieved nirvana—in order to alleviate the suffering of others. In order to continue his altruistic service to the world, Wolff resisted his strong inclination to retreat into the transcendent bliss of nondual consciousness.

His second realization resolved the tension between nondual consciousness and the phenomenal world. This realization resulted in a sense of perfect equilibrium between relative and ultimate levels of consciousness, without his being attached to either one. In this state of pristine awareness he no longer valued transcendent, nondual awareness over the experience of the phenomenal world, for he recognized that ultimately there was no difference between the two. Wolff called this realization "High Indifference," a complete resolution of tension between all opposites, very much in accordance with the writings of Nicholas of Cusa, which we will examine below. This entailed the complete transcendence of all distinctions, including between the transcendent and the relative. At this point all sense of personal identity had been relinquished, in terms of both a lower sense of an ego and the highest sense of a transcendent self.

During this awakening, which lasted several hours, Wolff felt a sense of identity with both a primordial "unlimited and abstract Space" and a "subject-object and self-analyzing consciousness" that had a "sort of point-presence within that Space."[6] This entailed a shift of consciousness away from individual identity toward a ground of consciousness that gives rise to the manifested world. Here he identified with a universal substrate in which he felt he knew the objects of the world through having become one with them, and this brought an extraordinary state of bliss. The parallel between his experience and philosophical reflections and the writings of the Neoplatonic Christian contemplatives is striking and suggests a convergence on universal truths that transcend any one time, place, or ideology.

CONVERGING COSMOLOGIES

Daniel C. Matt, one of the foremost contemporary scholars of Jewish mysticism, comments that if the scientific hypothesis of the multiple universes emerging one after another is correct, then the opening words of Genesis should be translated not as "In the beginning," but "In a beginning, God created heaven and earth." This actually represents a more literal rendering of the original Hebrew, *Be-Reshit*: "In a beginning."[7] According to the Jewish mystical tradition, the Kabbalah, "God" is a name we give to the oneness of all things. One name for God is Ein Sof, literally meaning "there is no end," suggesting the infinite nature of God. But an even deeper term is Ayin, referring to a divine nothingness that animates all things but is not contained by any of them. The entire physical universe emerges out of and is not other than this nothingness, which itself is filled with divine energy. This energy pervades all things but is concealed within them, for if it were not hidden, there could be no individual existence and everything would dissolve back into oneness, or the perfect symmetry of nothingness. The beginning of our universe, say the Jewish mystics, involved a "contraction," a withdrawal by which God allowed the physical universe to emerge. The vacuum created by this contraction became the womb of creation, but it was not really empty, for it retained a trace of the light of God. As a result, they believe that divine sparks exist in everything, and the spiritual challenge is to raise the sparks, to restore the world to God, to become aware that everything we experience is part of God's oneness. By devoting ourselves to spiritual practice, we arouse the sparks and thereby mend the broken symmetries of the cosmos.

Nicholas of Cusa's vision of the origins and evolution of the universe was remarkably similar to that of the Jewish mystics. Observing how, in a circumference carried to infinity, the straight and the curved line converge, he affirmed that in the infinity of God all opposites vanish and all distinctions fade into nothingness. In accordance with earlier Neoplatonic writings, he maintained that God is an absolute unity, transcending all opposites, but he becomes "contracted" into the multiple emanations of the world. Expressing a view remarkably similar to that of Origen, he wrote, "*Theos,* who is the beginning from which everything flows forth, the middle in which we move, and the end to which everything flows back again, is everything."[8] The universe, therefore, is permeated with the infinite potential of the divine, which is the essential nature of all things. Addressing this, Nicholas declared, "There is nothing outside you, but all things in you are not other than you. You teach me, Lord, how otherness, which is not in you, does not exist in itself, nor can it exist."[9]

Returning to the contemplative traditions of India, we once again find striking parallels to the contemplative cosmologies of Judaism and Christianity. According to the Advaita Vedanta school of Hinduism, discussed in chapter 10, the only ultimate reality is God (Brahman), devoid of conceivable characteristics. This ultimate dimension of the Divine manifests as God with characteristics, and creation occurs through a series of illusory, insubstantial manifestations. Likewise, the one True Self emanates into innumerable individual selves of every conscious being. The differentiations among these manifestations are illusory. Individual selves are therefore seen as mere "appearances" or "reflections" of the Self, like the sun reflected in rippling water. Likewise, God devoid of characteristics, which is pure consciousness, appears as the many objects in our experience. The Self, being nondifferent from the universe, cannot literally enter it, but metaphorically does so just as the sun "enters" the water by being perceived there in its reflection. The fact that ordinary people do not perceive the divine, illusory nature of all appearances is due to imperfections in their own minds, not in the appearances themselves. It is ignorance in the minds of living beings specifically, each grasping onto their own separate, independent, personal identity, that veils the natural awareness of God. When such ignorance is dispelled through spiritual practice, one recognizes one's own nature as identical to God.[10]

The Great Perfection tradition of Buddhism presents a view of cosmology with much in common with the preceding contemplative views. According to this tradition, the Primordial Buddha, known as Samantabhadra, is none other than the ultimate unity of the absolute space of phenomena, primordial consciousness, and primordial energy. This luminous space of consciousness causes the phenomenal world to appear, and it is none other than the nature of one's own mind, which is clear light.

Contemplatives of this tradition declare that the essential nature of each sentient being and the universe as a whole is infinite, luminous space, endowed with all the qualities of perfection. But the reality of all phenomena arising as displays of the all-pervasive awareness is obscured by ignorance.

Consequently, primordial consciousness, which utterly transcends all words and concepts—including the very notions of existence and nonexistence, one and many, and subject and object—is experientially reduced to the substrate together with the substrate consciousness. From that state of consciousness arises the sense of the self, or "I," which is apprehended as being "here," so the objective world seems to be "over there," thus establishing the appearance of space.

To relate this to the evolution of the universe, it is said that ignorance initially obscures the inner glow of one's innate, primordial consciousness of the absolute space of phenomena, which causes an external transference of its radiance. As the evolutionary process continues, the unity of primordial consciousness becomes differentiated into five different facets of awareness, which in turn emanate as the five physical elements of space, motion, heat, fluidity, and solidity, with each of these elements being present in all the others. Spiritual practice in this tradition is aimed at releasing the delusional sense of oneself as an independent being, fathoming the nature of one's own primordial consciousness, and fully manifesting the wisdom, compassion, and creative energy that is implicit in this ultimate dimension of reality.[11]

As a result of directing their attention outward into deep space, scientists have conceptually probed the origins and evolution of the universe back to the big bang. But since consciousness is invisible to all technological modes of observation and measurement, their vision of the cosmos is limited to its physical manifestations. By directing their attention inward, into the deep space of consciousness, contemplatives have experientially probed the origins and evolution of the universe back to its divine source, imbued with infinite consciousness and creative potential. Scientists and contemplatives alike have come to view our present world as a reflection of a greater perfection that temporarily lies hidden from view. For scientists this hypothesis remains a tantalizing, conceptual abstraction, but for contemplatives the experiential realization of the nature of that great perfection is the very meaning of life.

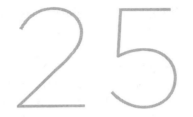

25

WHAT SHALL WE BECOME?

This book began with the question, who am I? to which we now turn once again. Insofar as we lead our lives mindlessly, simply reacting to situations without discerning mindfulness, we can indeed be likened to robots responding to stimuli based upon our neurochemical and genetic programs. Insofar as we follow our baser instincts, we can be regarded simply as animals, leading our lives under the influence of our genes, instincts, and emotions, with all our actions oriented toward survival, procreation, and the pursuit of mundane pleasures. In the grand scheme of things, human existence seems infinitesimally insignificant as we consider that we inhabit one planet in a solar system within a single galaxy with 100 billion stars within a known universe that includes 50 to 100 billion galaxies. When we consider our finite existence as biological organisms, the immensity of the universe is overwhelming.

Leading physicists cited in this book, however, have proposed that our role in the cosmos may not be as insignificant as it seems. The evolution of the universe from the big bang to the present day as we conceive and experience it has no objective, independent nature of its own. Rather, we choose the kind of world we inhabit as observer-participants. If this is true of the past and present, it is all the more true of our future. We are creating it with our every thought and action.

Judaism and Christianity insist there is more to human existence than can be understood with the methods of physics and biology. Humans are created in the image of God and have the capacity to evolve spiritually into more and more perfect reflections of our creator. In a similar spirit, Buddhism declares that all sentient beings, not only humans, are imbued with a buddha nature, and each one has the capacity to realize the perfect enlightenment of a buddha.

With our rapidly growing population, ravenous exploitation of the Earth's natural resources, and insatiable consumerism, humanity is swiftly and radically altering the biosphere in ways that are making it less and less conducive to human survival and flourishing. *We are on a trajectory of self-destruction, and since the human genome changes only one half of one percent every million years, it is impossible for us to evolve rapidly enough biologically to adapt to the environment we are shaping. For the sake of our very survival, let alone our flourishing as a species, we must now evolve spiritually through the cultivation of greater wisdom and insight into our own nature and our relation to the world around us.*

The meditations explained in this book, culminating in the Great Perfection, may be practiced by anyone, regardless of their beliefs. The purpose of presenting these theories and practices is not to convert people to Buddhism or any other religious faith but to suggest that they may be followed by anyone as a means to gain greater experiential insight into the nature of the mind and its relation to the rest of the world. By doing so, you may find that your way of life becomes more harmonious with those around you, that your mind becomes more balanced and peaceful, and that you experience a growing awareness of the inner resources of your own mind.

The insights you gain from such practices may then be integrated into your own belief system, whether you are Christian, Jewish, Muslim, Hindu, Taoist, Buddhist, agnostic, or hold to any other worldview. Most of the great contemplative traditions of the world have fallen into decline with the rise of modernity, but the time may now have come for people of different spiritual traditions to bring about a renaissance of their own contemplative heritages. By exploring contemplative practices, scientists too may broaden the horizons of their own disciplines—from physics to neuroscience—and thereby bring about the first great revolution in the mind sciences. The implications of such a revolution are bound to be far-reaching, challenging many of the current assumptions of physics and biology.

Every time one of us chooses to devote ourselves to contemplative practice, we change our world, shape our own future, and help to bring about a renewal of understanding and meaning in today's society. Through such practice, we may rediscover universal truths about our own identity, our potential for goodness, the nature of genuine happiness, and the role of consciousness in the universe. These truths have been revealed throughout history by the great wisdom traditions of human civilization, including religion, philosophy, and science. We are now poised for the greatest renaissance the world has seen, for the first time integrating the ancient and modern insights of the East and West. The time is ripe for humanity to take the next step in our spiritual evolution so that we can successfully rise to the challenges of today's world and flourish in the world to come.

NOTES

PART I: MEDITATION: WHERE IT STARTED AND HOW IT GOT HERE

1. WHO AM I?

1. D. M. Strong, trans., *The Udāna, or the Solemn Utterances of the Buddha* (Oxford: Pali Text Society, 1994), 68–69.

2. THE ORIGINS OF CONTEMPLATION

1. Josef Pieper, *Happiness and Contemplation,* trans. Richard and Clara Winston (Chicago: Henry Regnery Co., 1966), 73.
2. *Baudhāyana Śulbasūtra,* in T. A. Sarasvati Amma, *Geometry in Ancient and Medieval India* (Delhi: Motilal Banarsidass, 1979), 14–15.
3. *Metaphysics,* XIII, 6, 1080b16.
4. H. St. J. Thackeray, R. Marcus, A. Wikgren, and L. H. Feldman, trans., *Josephus* (Loeb Classical Library) (London: Heinemann, 1956).
5. Matthew 3:1–10.
6. Matthew 11:11.
7. Matthew 4:17.
8. Matthew 11:13–14; Matthew 17:12–14; Matthew 17:10–13; Luke 1:17.
9. 2 Kings 2:11.

10. See Thomas Merton, *Cassian and the Fathers: Initiation Into the Monastic Tradition* (Kalamazoo, Mich.: Cistercian Publications, 2005).

11. *Aṅguttara Nikāya* III:65; *Kalama Sutta: The Buddha's Charter of Free Inquiry,* trans. Soma Thera (Kandy, Sri Lanka: Buddhist Publication Society, 1981).

12. Bhikkhu Ñāṇamoli, *The Life of the Buddha According to the Pali Canon* (Kandy, Sri Lanka: Buddhist Publication Society, 1992), 10–29.

3. THE SCIENTIFIC EXTERNALIZATION OF MEDITATION

1. Dava Sobel, *Galileo's Daughter: A Historical Memoir of Science, Faith, and Love* (New York: Penguin, 2000), 326.

2. René Descartes, *Discourse on the Method of Rightly Conducting One's Reason and Seeking the Truth in the Sciences,* trans. Ian Maclean (New York: Oxford University Press, 2006).

3. René Descartes, *Discourse on Method and The Meditations* (London: Penguin, 1968), 122.

4. René Descartes, *A Discourse on Method; Meditations on the First Philosophy; Principles of Philosophy,* trans. John Veitch (London: Everyman, 1994), 1:66.

5. Ibid., 2:4.

6. Antonio Damasio, *The Feeling of What Happens: Body and Emotion in the Making of Consciousness* (New York: Harcourt, 1999), 321.

7. William James, "A Plea for Psychology as a Science," *Philosophical Review* 1 (1892): 146.

8. William James, *Some Problems of Philosophy: A Beginning of an Introduction to Philosophy* (London: Longmans, Green, 1911), 22–24.

9. William James, *The Principles of Psychology* (New York: Dover, 1950), I:1.

10. Ibid., I:185, 197–98.

11. Cf. Kurt Danziger, "The History of Introspection Reconsidered," *Journal of the History of the Behavioral Sciences* 16 (1980): 241–62.

12. Phillip H. Wiebe, "Religious Experience, Cognitive Science, and the Future of Religion," in *The Oxford Handbook of Religion and Science,* ed. Philip Clayton and Zachary Simpson (New York: Oxford University Press, 2006), 505.

13. John B. Watson, "Psychology as a Behaviorist Views It." *Psychological Review* 20 (1913): 158, 166.

14. Cf. Patricia Churchland and Terence J. Sejenowski, "Neural Representation and Neural Computation," in *Mind and Cognition: A Reader,* ed. William G. Lycan (Oxford: Blackwell, 1990), 227.

15. B. F. Skinner, *Science and Human Behavior* (New York: Macmillan, 1953).

16. John B. Watson, *Behaviorism* (1913; reprint, New York: Norton, 1970).

17. Christof Koch, *The Quest for Consciousness: A Neurobiological Approach* (Englewood, Colo.: Roberts and Co., 2004), 18–19.

18. Damasio, *The Feeling of What Happens,* 73, 169, 309, 311, 322–23.

19. Damasio, *The Feeling of What Happens,* 322.

1. Sharon Begley, *Train Your Mind, Change Your Brain: How a New Science Reveals Our Extraordinary Potential to Transform Ourselves* (New York: Ballantine, 2007).
2. Herbert Benson, *The Relaxation Response* (New York: Avon, 1976).
3. C. R. MacLean, et al., "Effects of the Transcendental Meditation Program on Adaptive Mechanisms: Changes in Hormone Levels and Responses to Stress After Four Months of Practice," *Psychoneuroendocrinology* 22, no. 4 (May 1997): 277–95.
4. R. Bonadonna, "Meditation's Impact on Chronic Illness," *Holistic Nursing Practice* 17, no. 6 (Nov.–Dec. 2003): 309–19.
5. Anne Bruce and Betty Davies, "Mindfulness in Hospice Care: Practicing Meditation-in-Action," *Qualitative Health Research* 15, no. 10 (2005): 1329–1344. See also Bruce A. Davies, "Mindfulness in Hospice Care: Practicing Meditation-in-Action," *Qualitative Health Research* 15, no. 10 (Dec. 2005): 1329–1344; T. A. Richards, D. Oman, J. Hedberg, C. E. Thoresen, and J. Bowden, "A Qualitative Examination of a Spiritually-Based Intervention and Self-Management in the Workplace," *Nursing Science Quarterly* 19, no. 3 (July 2006): 231–39; Denise Barham, "The Last 48 Hours of Life: A Case Study of Symptom Control for a Patient Taking a Buddhist Approach to Dying," *International Journal of Palliative Nursing* 9, no. 6 (June 2003): 245; Maria Wasner, Christine Longaker, Martin Johannes Fegg, and Gian Domenico Borasio, "Effects of Spiritual Care Training for Palliative Care Professionals," *Palliative Medicine* 19 (2005): 99–104.
6. S. Bishop, "What Do We Really Know About Mindfulness-Based Stress Reduction?" *Psychosomatic Medicine* 64 (2002): 71.
7. Daniel Goleman, ed., *Healing Emotions: Conversations with the Dalai Lama on Mindfulness, Emotions, and Health* (Boston: Shambhala, 1997).
8. Zindel V. Segal, et al., *Mindfulness-Based Cognitive Therapy for Depression: A New Approach to Preventing Relapse* (New York: Guilford, 2002); Zindel V. Segal, et al., "Mindfulness-Based Cognitive Therapy: Theoretical Rationale and Empirical Status," in *Mindfulness and Acceptance: Expanding the Cognitive-Behavioral Tradition,* ed. S. C. Hayes et al. (New York: Guilford, 2004); John D. Teasdale et al., "Prevention of Relapse/Recurrence in Major Depression by Mindfulness-Based Cognitive Therapy," *Journal of Consulting and Clinical Psychology* 68, no. 4 (Aug. 2000): 615–23; M. Speca et al., "A Randomized Wait-List Controlled Clinical Trial: The Effect of a Mindfulness Meditation-Based Stress Reduction Program on Mood and Symptoms of Stress in Cancer Outpatients," *Psychosomatic Medicine* 62, no. 5 (Sept.–Oct. 2000): 613–22; G. Bogart, "The Use of Meditation in Psychotherapy: A Review of the Literature," *American Journal of Psychotherapy* 45, no. 3 (July 1991): 383–412.
9. See http://www.investigatingthemind.org/.
10. Richard J. Davidson et al., "Alterations in Brain and Immune Function Produced by Mindfulness Meditation," *Psychosomatic Medicine* 65, no. 4 (July–Aug. 2003): 564–70.
11. Antoine Lutz, Laurence L. Greischar, Nancy B. Rawlings, Matthieu Ricard, and Richard J. Davidson, "Long-Term Meditators Self-Induce High-Amplitude Gamma Synchrony During

Mental Practice," *Proceedings of the National Academy of Science* 101, no. 46 (Nov. 16, 2004): 16369–16373.

12. See http://lazar-meditation-research.info/lazar.html.

13. S. W. Lazar, C. E. Kerr, R. H. Wasserman, J. R. Gray, D. N. Greve, M. T. Treadway, M. Mc-Garvey, B. T. Quinn, J. A. Dusek, H. Benson, S. L. Rauch, C. I. Moore, and B. Fischl, "Meditation Experience Is Associated with Increased Cortical Thickness," *Neuroreport* 16 (2005): 893–97.

14. M. R. Rueda, M. K. Rothbart, B. D. McCandliss, L. Saccomanno, and M. I. Posner, *Proceedings of the National Academy of Science USA* 102 (2005): 14931–14936; Karla Homboe and Mark H. Johnson, "Educating Executive Attention," *Proceedings of the National Academy of Science* 102, no. 41 (Oct. 11, 2005): 14479–14480.

15. Amishi P. Jha, Jason Krompinger, and Michael J. Baime, "Mindfulness Training Modifies Subsystems of Attention," *Cognitive, Affective, and Behavioral Neuroscience* 7, no. 2 (2007): 109–19; Heleen A. Slagter, Antoine Lutz, Lawrence L. Greischar, Andrew D. Francis, Sander Nieuwenhuls, James M. Davis, and Richard J. Davidson, "Mental Training Affects Distribution of Limited Brain Resources," *Public Library of Science Biology* 5, no. 6 (June 2007): 1–8; Yi-Yuan Tang, Yinghua Ma, Junhong Wang, Yaxin Fan, Shigang Feng, Qilin Lu, Qingbao Yu, Danni Sui, Mary K. Rothbart, Ming Fan, and Michael I. Posner, "Short-Term Meditation Training Improves Attention and Self-Regulation," *PNAS Early Edition* (August 16, 2007); www.pnas.org/cgi/doi/10.1073/pnas.0707678104.

16. Paul Ekman, Richard J. Davidson, Matthieu Ricard, and B. Alan Wallace, "Buddhist and Psychological Perspectives on Emotions and Well-Being," *Current Directions in Psychology* 14, no. 2 (2005): 59–63; B. Alan Wallace and Shauna Shapiro, "Mental Balance and Well-Being: Building Bridges Between Buddhism and Western Psychology," *American Psychologist* 161, no. 7 (Oct. 2006): 690–701; http://www.sbinstitute.com/mentalbalance.pdf.

17. Daniel Goleman, ed., *Destructive Emotions: A Scientific Dialogue with the Dalai Lama* (New York: Bantam Doubleday, 2002).

18. Paul Ekman, *Emotions Revealed: Recognizing Faces and Feelings to Improve Communication and Emotional Life* (New York: Times Books, 2003), 39–40.

19. Katherine Ellison, "Mastering Your Own Mind," *Psychology Today* (Oct. 2006); http://www.psychologytoday.com (click on "Mastering Your Own Mind").

20. Louis Sahagun, "The Dalai Lama Has It—but Just What Is 'It'?" *Los Angeles Times*, Dec. 9, 2006, B2.

21. The Dalai Lama, *Freedom in Exile: The Autobiography of the Dalai Lama* (New York: Harper-Collins, 1990).

6. THEORY: COMING TO OUR SENSES

1. Saint Maximus the Confessor, Scholia on *The Divine Names*, PG 4, 208 C. Cited in Martin Laird, *Into the Silent Land: A Guide to the Practice of Christian Contemplation* (New York: Oxford University Press, 2006), 37. See John 4:28. "God is spirit." Cited in Olivier Clément,

The Roots of Christian Mysticism, trans. T. Berkeley (London: New City Press, 1993), 33. The Greek word translated as "spirit" is *pneuma,* which can also mean "breath."

2. Martin Laird, *Into the Silent Land: A Guide to the Practice of Christian Contemplation* (New York: Oxford University Press, 2006), 34–45.

3. Saint Symeon the New Theologian, "The Three Methods of Prayer," in *The Philokalia: The Complete Text,* trans. G.E.H. Palmer, Philip Sherrard, and Kallistos Ware (London: Faber and Faber, 1995), IV:67–75.

4. Saint Gregory Palamas, "In Defense of Those Who Devoutly Practice a Life of Stillness," in *The Philokalia: The Complete Text,* trans. G.E.H. Palmer, Philip Sherrard, and Kallistos Ware (London: Faber and Faber, 1995), IV:337.

5. Ibid.

6. Saint John of the Cross, *The Spiritual Canticle,* in *The Collected Works of St. John of the Cross,* trans. K. Kavanaugh and R. Rodriguez (Washington, D.C.: Institute of Carmelite Studies, 1979), Red A., str. 38.

7. PRACTICE: THE UNION OF STILLNESS AND MOTION

1. Padmasambhava, *Natural Liberation: Padmasambhava's Teachings on the Six Bardos,* commentary by Gyatrul Rinpoche, trans. B. Alan Wallace (Boston: Wisdom, 1998), 90–92.

8. THEORY: KNOWING AND HEALING THE MIND

1. Romans 1:28–32.

2. Romans 2:6, 2:8, 3:10, 3:22.

3. P. T. Raju, *Structural Depths of Indian Thought* (Albany: State University of New York Press, 1985), chap. 3.

4. Sigmund Freud, *Civilization and Its Discontents,* trans. and ed. James Strachey (New York: Norton, 1961), 33.

5. Ibid., 24–25.

6. Ibid., 33.

7. Daniel M. Wegner, *The Illusion of Conscious Will* (Cambridge, Mass.: MIT Press, 2003).

8. Hakwan C. Lau, Robert D. Rogers, and Richard E. Passingham, "Manipulating the Experienced Onset of Intention After Action Execution," *Journal of Cognitive Neuroscience* 19, no. 1 (Jan. 2007): 81–90.

9. Andrew F. Leuchter et al., "Changes in Brain Function of Depressed Subjects During Treatment with Placebo," *American Journal of Psychiatry* 159 (2002): 122–29.

10. John Burnaby, *Amor Dei: A Study of the Religion of St. Augustine* (1938; reprint, Norwich, England: Canterbury Press, 1991), 57.

11. *The Dhammapada,* ed. Nikunja Vihari Banerjee (New Delhi: Munshiram Manoharlal Publishers, 1989), I:1.

12. Sermon 8, "On the Third Commandment," cited in Martin Laird, *Into the Silent Land: A Guide to the Practice of Christian Contemplation* (New York: Oxford University Press, 2006), 52.

13. Evagrius, *The Praktikos*, chap. 50, in *The Praktikos and Chapters on Prayer*, trans. J. Bamberger (Kalamazoo, Mich.: Cistercian Publications, 1981), 29–30.

14. Ibid., chap. 54, 31.

15. Kallistos Ware, "Ways of Prayer and Contemplation: I. Eastern," in *Christian Spirituality: Origins to the Twelfth Century*, ed. Bernard McGinn and John Meyendorff (New York: Crossroad, 1985), 398.

16. Thomas Keating, *Open Mind, Open Heart: The Contemplative Dimension of the Gospel* (New York: Crossroad, 2001), 93–107.

17. Laird, *Into the Silent Land*, 63.

18. *Sutta Nipāta* 47.10, cited in Collett Cox, "Mindfulness and Memory: The Scope of *Smṛti* from Early Buddhism to the Sarvāstivādin Abhidharma," in *In the Mirror or Memory: Reflections on Mindfulness and Remembrance in Indian and Tibetan Buddhism*, ed. Janet Gyatso (Albany: State University of New York Press, 1992), 71.

19. *Sutta Nipāta* 47.8, cited in Cox, "Mindfulness and Memory," 71.

20. Karma Chagmé, *A Spacious Path to Freedom: Practical Instructions on the Union of Mahāmudrā and Atiyoga*, commentary by Gyatrul Rinpoche, trans. B. Alan Wallace (Ithaca, N.Y.: Snow Lion, 1998), 80.

21. Panchen Lozang Chökyi Gyaltsen, "Sems gnas pa'i thabs" section of his *dGe ldan bKa' brgyud rin po che'i bka' srol phyag rgya chen po'i rtsa ba rgyas par bshad pa yang gsal sgron me*, cited in B. Alan Wallace, *Balancing the Mind: A Tibetan Buddhist Approach to Refining Attention* (Ithaca, N.Y.: Snow Lion, 2005), 174; cf. Panchen Lozang Chökyi Gyaltsen, *The Great Seal of Voidness*, in *The Mahāmudrā Eliminating the Darkness of Ignorance*, trans. Alex Berzin (Dharamsala: Library of Tibetan Works and Archives, 1978); Geshe Rabten, *Echoes of Voidness*, trans. and ed. Stephen Batchelor (London: Wisdom, 1986), 113–28; H. H. the Dalai Lama and Alex Berzin, *The Gelug/Kagyü Tradition of Mahamudra* (Ithaca, N.Y.: Snow Lion, 1997).

22. Düdjom Lingpa, *The Vajra Essence: From the Matrix of Pure Appearances and Primordial Consciousness, a Tantra on the Self-Originating Nature of Existence*, trans. B. Alan Wallace (Alameda, Calif.: Mirror of Wisdom, 2004), 19.

23. Ibid.

24. Ibid., 20.

25. Ibid., 26–27.

26. Burnaby, *Amor Dei*, 47–48.

27. Laird, *Into the Silent Land*, 41.

28. Maurice Walshe, *The Long Discourses of the Buddha: A Translation of the Dīgha Nikāya* (Somerville, Mass.: Wisdom, 1995), 245.

29. René Descartes, *A Discourse on Method; Meditations on the First Philosophy; Principles of Philosophy*, trans. John Veitch (London: Everyman, 1994), part IV.

30. Mark Epstein, *Thoughts Without a Thinker: Psychotherapy from a Buddhist Perspective* (New York: Basic Books, 1995).

31. D. K. Nauriyal, ed., *Buddhist Thought and Applied Psychology: Transcending the Boundaries* (London: Routledge-Curzon, 2006); Mark Unno, ed., *Buddhism and Psychotherapy Across Cultures: Essays on Theories and Practices* (Boston: Wisdom, 2006).

32. Scott R. Bishop et al., "Mindfulness: A Proposed Operational Definition," *Clinical Psychology: Science and Practice* 11, no. 3 (Fall 2004): 232.

33. *Saṃyutta-Nikāya* V:197–98; *Sutta Nipāta* 48.9.

34. *Milindapañha* 37–38; cf. Rupert M. L. Gethin, *The Buddhist Path to Awakening* (Oxford: Oneworld, 2001), 36–44.

35. Buddhaghosa, *The Path of Purification*, trans. Ñāṇamoli Bhikkhu (Kandy, Sri Lanka: Buddhist Publication Society, 1979), XIV:141.

36. *Dīgha Nikāya* III:269 and *Aṅguttara Nikāya* V:30.

37. *Aṅguttara Nikāya* IV:385, *Aṅguttara Nikāya* IV:339, and *Aṅguttara Nikāya* V:107, as well as *Theragāthā* 359 and 446, all refer to the controlling influence of mindfulness on the mind.

38. *Papañcasūdanī* (commentary to the *Majjhima Nikāya*) I:292, 243; *Ps- purāṇaṭīkā* (commentary to the *Majjhima Nikāya*) I:363, cited in Anālayo, *Satipaṭṭhāna: The Direct Path to Realization* (Birmingham, England: Windhorse, 2006), 235.

39. *Sutta Nipāta* 47.35; Śāntideva, *A Guide to the Bodhisattva Way of Life*, trans. Vesna A. Wallace and B. Alan Wallace (Ithaca, N.Y.: Snow Lion, 1997), V:108.

40. Buddhaghosa, *The Path of Purification*, IV:172.

41. *Dantabhūmi Sutta* (*Majjhima Nikāya* 125).

42. Evan Thompson, *Mind in Life: Biology, Phenomenology, and the Sciences of Mind* (Cambridge, Mass.: Belknap Press, 2007).

43. Christof Koch, *The Quest for Consciousness: A Neurobiological Approach* (Englewood, Colo.: Roberts and Co., 2004), 18–19.

44. William James, *The Principles of Psychology* (1890; reprint, New York: Dover, 1950), I:190.

10. THEORY: EXPLORING THE NATURE OF CONSCIOUSNESS

1. Heychios, *On Watchfulness and Holiness*, chap. 14, in *The Philokalia*, trans. G. Palmer, P. Sherrard, and K. Ware (London: Faber and Faber, 1979), I:vs. 5.

2. Ibid., vs. 132; Heychios, *On Watchfulness*, chap. 7, in *The Philokalia*, I:163.

3. Saint Symeon the New Theologian, "The Three Methods of Prayer," in *The Philokalia: The Complete Text*, trans. G.E.H. Palmer, Philip Sherrard, and Kallistos Ware (London: Faber and Faber, 1995), IV:72.

4. Sister Benedicta Ward, *The Sayings of the Desert Fathers: The Alphabetical Collection*, 2nd ed. (London: Oxford University Press, 1981), 139.

5. Saint Gregory Palamas, "In Defense of Those Who Devoutly Practice a Life of Stillness," in *The Philokalia: The Complete Text*, trans. G.E.H. Palmer, Philip Sherrard, and Kallistos Ware (London: Faber and Faber, 1995), IV:334.

6. Saint Gregory Palamas, *The Triads*, ed. John Meyendorff, trans. Nicholas Gendle (New York: Paulist Press, 1983), I, ii, 3.

7. Theophan cited in Igumen Chariton of Valamo, *The Art of Prayer*, trans. E. Kadloubovsky and E. Palmer (London: Faber and Faber, 1966), 183.

8. Martin Laird, *Into the Silent Land: A Guide to the Practice of Christian Contemplation* (New York: Oxford University Press, 2006), 92.

9. William James, "Does Consciousness Exist?" in *The Writings of William James*, ed. John J. McDermott (1904; reprint, Chicago: University of Chicago Press, 1977), 177–78; "The Notion of Consciousness," in *The Writings of William James*, 184–94.

10. William James, "A Plea for Psychology as a Science," *Philosophical Review* 1 (1892): 146.

11. William James, *Some Problems of Philosophy: A Beginning of an Introduction to Philosophy* (London: Longmans, Green, 1911), 22–24.

12. Cited in Dava Sobel, *Galileo's Daughter: A Historical Memoir of Science, Faith, and Love* (New York: Penguin, 2000), 326.

13. Daniel Dennett, *Content and Consciousness* (New York: Routledge & Kegan Paul, 1969), 40.

14. Ibid., 21–22.

15. Imants Barušs, *Science as Spiritual Practice* (Charlottesville, Va.: Imprint Academic, 2007), 93–117.

16. Bina Gupta, *The Disinterested Witness: A Fragment of Advaita Vedānta Phenomenology* (Evanston, Ill. Northwestern University Press, 1998), 3–4.

17. http://www.om-guru.com/html/saints/wolff.html.

18. Ron Leonard, *The Transcendent Philosophy of Franklin Merrell-Wolff* (Albany: State University of New York Press, 1999), 49.

19. Franklin Merrell-Wolff, *Mathematics, Philosophy, and Yoga: A Lecture Series Presented at the Los Olivos Conference Room in Phoenix, Arizona in 1966* (Phoenix, Ariz.: Phoenix Philosophical Press, 1995), 50–51.

20. Franklin Merrell-Wolff, *Franklin Merrell-Wolff's Experience and Philosophy* (Albany: State University of New York Press, 2003), 265.

21. Ibid., 269.

22. *Aṅguttara Nikāya* V.60.

23. *Majjhima Nikāya* 77.

24. Padmasambhava, *Natural Liberation: Padmasambhava's Teachings on the Six Bardos*, commentary by Gyatrul Rinpoche, trans. B. Alan Wallace (Boston: Wisdom, 1998), 107.

25. Shabkar Tsokdrug Rangdröl, *The Flight of the Garuda*, in *The Flight of the Garuda*, trans. Erik Pema Kunsang, 4th ed. (Kathmandu: Rangjung Yeshe Publications, 1993), 21–22.

26. Karma Chagmé, *A Spacious Path to Freedom: Practical Instructions on the Union of Mahāmudrā and Atiyoga*, commentary by Gyatrul Rinpoche, trans. B. Alan Wallace (Ithaca, N.Y.: Snow Lion, 1998), 80.

27. His citation is from the "Sems gnas pa'i thabs" section of Panchen Lozang Chökyi Gyaltsen's *dGe ldan bKa' brgyud rin po che'i bka' srol phyag rgya chen po'i rtsa ba rgyas par bshad pa yang gsal sgron me.Phyag rgya chen po'i rtsa ba* (Asian Classics Input Project, Source CD, Release A, S5939F.ACT, 1993).

28. Sobel, *Galileo's Daughter*, 32–33.

29. Saint Augustine, *The Literal Meaning of Genesis*, trans. John Hammond Taylor (New York: Newman Press, 1982), xii, 26, 53.

30. Bhikkhu Sujato, *A History of Mindfulness: How Insight Worsted Tranquility in the Satipatthana Sutta* (Taipei: The Corporate Body of the Buddha Educational Foundation, 2005), 140.

31. *Sutta Nipāta Sagāthā Vagga* verse 269, *Aṅguttara Nikāya* (4) 449–51.

32. *Majjhima Nikāya* I:301.

33. *Majjhima Nikāya* I:122; I:214; *The Dhammapada*, ed. Nikunja Vihari Banerjee (New Delhi: Munshiram Manoharlal Publishers, 1989), 326.

34. Buddhaghosa, *The Path of Purification*, trans. Ñāṇamoli Bhikkhu (Kandy, Sri Lanka: Buddhist Publication Society, 1979), 126.

35. *Saṃyutta Nikāya* IV:263.

36. *Majjhima Nikāya* I:463; *Dīgha Nikāya* I:75.

37. *Aṅguttara Nikāya* III:63; *Majjhima Nikāya* I:323.

38. *Dīgha Nikāya* II:313; *Saṃyutta Nikāya* V:10.

39. Asaṅga, *Abhidharmasamuccaya*, ed. Pralhad Pradhan (Santiniketan: Visva-Bharati, 1950), 75.21; Tsong-kha-pa, *The Great Treatise on the Stages of the Path to Enlightenment* (Ithaca, N.Y.: Snow Lion, 2002), 3:25, 95; B. Alan Wallace, *Balancing the Mind: A Tibetan Buddhist Approach to Refining Attention* (Ithaca, N.Y.: Snow Lion, 2005), 214.

11. PRACTICE: PROBING THE NATURE OF THE OBSERVER

1. Padmasambhava, *Natural Liberation: Padmasambhava's Teachings on the Six Bardos*, commentary by Gyatrul Rinpoche, trans. B. Alan Wallace (Boston: Wisdom, 1998), 105.

12. THEORY: THE GROUND STATE OF CONSCIOUSNESS

1. *Saṃyutta Nikāya* V:152; *Majjhima Nikāya* I:360.

2. John R. Searle, *Consciousness and Language* (Cambridge: Cambridge University Press, 2002), 35.

3. Peter Harvey, *The Selfless Mind: Personality, Consciousness and Nirvana in Early Buddhism* (Surrey: Curzon Press, 1995), 173.

4. *Kathāvatthu* 615; *Milindapañha* 299–300.

5. This is the view of the Mahāsāṅghika school, described in A. Bareau, *Les Sectes Bouddhiques du Petit Véhicule* (Paris: EFEO, 1955), 72.

6. Asaṅga, *Abhidharmasamuccaya*, ed. Pralhad Pradhan (Santiniketan: Visva-Bharati, 1950), 4–10.

7. Tao Jiang, *Yogācāra Buddhism and Modern Psychology on the Subliminal Mind*, Society for Asian and Comparative Philosophy Monographs, No. 21 (Honolulu: University of Hawaii Press, 2006); http://www.uhpress.hawaii.edu/books/jiang-intro.pdf.

8. B. Alan Wallace, *The Attention Revolution: Unlocking the Power of the Focused Mind* (Boston: Wisdom, 2006), 155–65.

9. Düdjom Lingpa, *The Vajra Essence: From the Matrix of Pure Appearances and Primordial Consciousness, a Tantra on the Self-Originating Nature of Existence,* trans. B. Alan Wallace (Alameda, Calif.: Mirror of Wisdom, 2004), 252–53.

10. Ibid., 92.

11. See the "Sems gnas pa'i thabs" section of his *dGe ldan bKa' brgyud rin po che'i bka' srol phyag rgya chen po'i rtsa ba rgyas par bshad pa yang gsal sgron me* [*Phyag rgya chen po'i rtsa ba*] (Asian Classics Input Project, Source CD, Release A, S5939F.ACT, 1993).

12. Düdjom Lingpa, *The Vajra Essence*, 30, 364–65.

13. B. Alan Wallace, "Vacuum States of Consciousness: A Tibetan Buddhist View," in *Buddhist Thought and Applied Psychology: Transcending the Boundaries,* ed. D. K. Nauriyal (London: Routledge-Curzon, 2006), 112–21.

14. The nature and role of the *jiva* is explained by Puṇḍarīka in *The Stainless Light* (*Vimalaprabhā*), the primary commentary to the *Kālacakratantra.*

15. Düdjom Lingpa, *The Vajra Essence*, 252.

16. Arthur Zajonc, ed., *The New Physics and Cosmology: Dialogues with the Dalai Lama* (New York: Oxford University Press, 2004), 92; H.H. the Dalai Lama, *The Universe in a Single Atom: The Convergence of Science and Spirituality* (New York: Morgan Road, 2005).

17. B. Alan Wallace, *Hidden Dimensions: The Unification of Physics and Consciousness* (New York: Columbia University Press, 2007), 50–69.

18. B. Alan Wallace, *Contemplative Science: Where Buddhism and Neuroscience Converge* (New York: Columbia University Press), 14–19.

19. William James, *Essays in Religion and Morality* (Cambridge, Mass.: Harvard University Press, 1989), 85–86.

14. THEORY: CONSCIOUSNESS WITHOUT BEGINNING OR END

1. Plato, *Phaedo,* in *The Collected Dialogues of Plato,* ed. Edith Hamilton and Huntington Cairns, trans. Hugh Tredennick, Bollingen Series LXXI (Princeton: Princeton University Press, 1961), 80–82.

2. Ibid., 81 a.

3. Ibid., 81 c–d.

4. *Bṛhadāraṇyaka Upaniṣad* IV.4.2; K. Werner, "Indian Concepts of Human Personality in Relation to the Doctrine of the Soul," *Journal of the Royal Asiatic Society* 1 (1988): 73–97, 82–83.

5. *Dīgha Nikāya* II:334.

6. *Dīgha Nikāya* I:77; *Dīgha Nikāya* II:62–63; *The Dhammapada,* ed. Nikunja Vihari Banerjee (New Delhi: Munshiram Manoharlal Publishers, 1989), 37; *Theragāthā* 355; Peter Harvey, "The Mind-Body Relationship in Pāli Buddhism—a Philosophical Investigation," *Asian Philosophy* 3 (1) (1993): 29–41.

7. Buddhaghosa, *The Path of Purification,* trans. Ñāṇamoli Bhikkhu (Kandy, Sri Lanka: Buddhist Publication Society, 1979), XVII.

8. *Saṃyutta Nikāya* IV:399–400.

9. *Aṅguttara Nikāya* II:134.

10. *Dīgha Nikāya* I:83; *Majjhima Nikāya* I:261–62.

11. Harvey, *The Selfless Mind,* 103.

12. The Harris Poll, July 17–21, 1998.

13. Matthew 22:23.

14. John 3:3.

15. Matthew 11:11–15; 17:10–13.

16. Origen, de Principiis; http://www.iep.utm.edu/o/origen.htm.

17. Cf. I Corinthians 15:28.

18. Saint Augustine, *The Free Choice of the Will* (391), trans. Francis E. Tourscher (Philadelphia: The Peter Reilly Co., 1937), bk. III, chs. 20–21.

19. Ibid., 379.

20. Gershom Scholem, ed., *Zohar, The Book of Splendor: Basic Readings from the Kabbalah* (New York: Schocken, 1995).

21. *Majjhima Nikāya* I:265–66.

22. *Aṅguttara Nikāya* II:183, V:336.

23. Yuho Yokoi, *Zen Master Dogen: An Introduction with Selected Writings* (New York: Weatherhill, 1976).

24. For a fascinating, well-researched discussion of the closed-mindedness of the scientific community to empirical evidence that challenges their materialistic assumptions, see Deborah Blum, *Ghost Hunters: William James and the Search for Scientific Proof of Life After Death* (New York: Penguin, 2006).

25. For a partial list of his articles published in scientific journals, see http://www.healthsystem .virginia.edu/internet/personalitystudies/publications.cfm.

26. Ian Stevenson, M.D., *Reincarnation and Biology: A Contribution to the Etiology of Birthmarks and Birth Defects* (New York: Praeger, 1997); Ian Stevenson, M.D., *Where Reincarnation and Biology Intersect* (New York: Praeger, 1997); Jim Tucker, *Life Before Life: A Scientific Investigation of Children's Memories of Previous Lives* (New York: St. Martin's Press, 2005); Edward F. Kelly, Emily Williams Kelly, Adam Crabtree, Alan Gauld, Michael Grosso, and Bruce Greyson, *Irreducible Mind: Toward a Psychology for the 21st Century* (Lanham, Md.: Rowman & Littlefield, 2007), 232–36.

27. Stevenson, *Reincarnation and Biology,* 1:455–67.

28. Stevenson, *Reincarnation and Biology,* 1:933–34.

29. Stevenson, *Reincarnation and Biology,* 2:2083–2092.

30. Karma Thinley, *History of 16 Karmapas* (Boston: Shambhala, 2001).

31. Poonam Sharma and Jim B. Tucker, "Cases of the Reincarnation Type with Memories from the Intermission Between Lives," *Journal of Near-Death Studies* 23 (2) (Winter 2004): 116.

32. For a full account of this occurrence, see Michael Sabom, *Light and Death: One Doctor's Fascinating Account of Near-Death Experiences* (Grand Rapids, Mich.: Zondervan, 1998). See

also the National Geographic Channel documentary *I Came Back from the Dead*, aired on July 29, 2008.

33. Harald Atmanspacher and Hans Primas, "The Hidden Side of Wolfgang Pauli," *Journal of Consciousness Studies* 3 (1996): 112–26.

34. Buddhaghosa, *The Path of Purification*, XIII:13–120.

35. Pa-Auk Tawya Sayadaw, *Knowing and Seeing* (Kuala Lumpur, Malaysia: WAVE Publications, 2003), 229–33; Geshe Gedün Lodrö, *Walking Through Walls: A Presentation of Tibetan Meditation*, trans. and ed. Jeffrey Hopkins (Ithaca, N.Y.: Snow Lion, 1992), 287–88.

36. Private conversation with Yangthang Rinpoche in Ojai, California, December 4, 2006.

37. Carrie Peyton Dahlberg, "Meditation Study Aims to Leap Over Mental Barriers," *Sacramento Bee*, November 29, 2004; http://www.sacbee.com/content/news/story/11608921p-12498535c .html; http://www.sbinstitute.com/Shamathatalk.html.

38. Stephen LaBerge and Howard Rheingold, *Exploring the World of Lucid Dreaming* (New York: Ballantine, 1990).

39. Plato, *The Republic*, trans. R. E. Allen (New Haven: Yale University Press, 2006), book X; http://classics.mit.edu/Plato/republic.11.x.html.

40. B. Alan Wallace, *Genuine Happiness: Meditation as the Path to Fulfillment* (Hoboken, N.J.: Wiley, 2005), chs. 12 and 13; Stephen LaBerge, "Lucid Dreaming and the Yoga of the Dream State: A Psychophysiological Perspective," in *Buddhism and Science: Breaking New Ground*, ed. B. Alan Wallace (New York: Columbia University Press, 2003), 233–58.

41. Stevenson, *Where Reincarnation and Biology Intersect*, ch. 6.

42. L. A. Finelli, P. Achermann, and A. Borbély, "Individual Fingerprints in Human Sleep EEG Topography." *Neuropsychopharmacology* 25 (2001): S57–S62; L. De Gennaro, M. Ferrara, F. Vecchio, G. Curcio, and M. Bertini, "An Electroencephalographic Fingerprint of Human Sleep," *NeuroImage* 26 (2005): 114–22; J. Buckelmüller, H. P. Landolt, H. H. Stassen, and P. Achermann, "Trait-like Individual Differences in the Human Sleep Electroencephalogram," *Neuroscience* 138 (2006): 351–56; G. Tinguely, L. A. Finelli, H. P. Landolt, A. A. Borbély, and P. Achermann, "Functional EEG Topography in Sleep and Waking: State-Dependent and State-Independent Features," *NeuroImage* 32 (2006): 283–92.

15. PRACTICE: RESTING IN THE STILLNESS OF AWARENESS

1. Padmasambhava, *Natural Liberation: Padmasambhava's Teachings on the Six Bardos*, commentary by Gyatrul Rinpoche, trans. B. Alan Wallace (Boston: Wisdom, 1998), 105–9.

16. THEORY: WORLDS OF SKEPTICISM

1. http://www.msnbc.msn.com/id/18825863/.

2. Sharon Begley, "Know Thyself—Man, Rat or Bot," *Newsweek*, April 23, 2007; http://www .msnbc.msn.com/id/18108859/site/newsweek/.

3. Robin Marantz Henig, "The Real Transformers," *New York Times,* July 29, 2007; http://www .nytimes.com/2007/07/29/magazine/29robots-t.html?_r=1&adxnnl=1&oref=slogin&adxnnl x=1185711249-XL9nqJdFDjGpK4ck3uvoxQ.

4. Ibid.

5. *Anguttara Nikāya* III:65.

6. B. F. Skinner, *About Behaviorism* (New York: Knopf, 1974), 31.

7. Ibid., 207–208.

8. Skinner, *About Behaviorism,* 30.

9. Skinner, *About Behaviorism,* 216.

10. Daniel C. Dennett, "The Fantasy of First-Person Science" (a written version of a debate with David Chalmers, held at Northwestern University, Evanston, Ill., February 15, 2001, supplemented by an e-mail debate with Alvin Goldman) (Third Draft March 1, 2001); http://ase .tufts.edu/cogstud/papers/chalmersdeb3dft.htm; Daniel C. Dennett, *Consciousness Explained* (Boston: Little, Brown, 1991).

11. Daniel C. Dennett, *Breaking the Spell: Religion as a Natural Phenomenon* (New York: Viking, 2006), 306.

12. John R. Searle, *The Rediscovery of the Mind* (Cambridge, Mass.: MIT Press, 1994), 95.

13. Ibid., 20.

14. Searle, *The Rediscovery of the Mind,* 142–43.

15. Searle, *The Rediscovery of the Mind,* 97, 99, 144.

16. Skinner, *About Behaviorism,* 211.

17. Victor A. F. Lamme, "Towards a True Neural Stance on Consciousness," *TRENDS in Cognitive Sciences* 10, no. 11 (Nov. 2006): 494.

18. Martin Buber, *Between Man and Man,* trans. Ronald Gregor Smith (New York: Macmillan, 1948), 184.

19. Lee Silver, "Life 2.0," *Newsweek International,* June 4, 2007; http://www.msnbc.msn .com/id/18882828/site/newsweek/.

20. Eric R. Kandel, *In Search of Memory: The Emergence of a New Science of Mind* (New York: Norton, 2007), 376.

21q. Allison L. Foote and Jonathan D. Crystal, "Metacognition in the Rat," *Current Biology* 17 (March 20, 2007): 551–55.

22. Sharon Begley, "Know Thyself—Man, Rat or Bot." *Newsweek,* April 23, 2007; http://www .msnbc.msn.com/id/18108859/site/newsweek/

23. Richard P. Feynman, *The Character of Physical Law* (Cambridge, Mass.: MIT Press, 1965), 127, 148, 158.

17. PRACTICE: THE EMPTINESS OF MIND

1. Padmasambhava, *Natural Liberation: Padmasambhava's Teachings on the Six Bardos,* commentary by Gyatrul Rinpoche, trans. B. Alan Wallace (Boston: Wisdom, 1998), 116–20.

18. THEORY: THE PARTICIPATORY WORLDS OF BUDDHISM

1. *Paṭisambhidāmagga* II:232; *Papañcasdanūdanī* I:242 (commentary to *Majjhima Nikāya*).

2. *Saṃyutta Nikāya* IV:400.

3. Anālayo Bhikkhu, *Satipaṭṭhāna: The Direct Path to Realization* (Birmingham, England: Windhorse, 2006); Gen Lamrimpa, *Realizing Emptiness: Madhyamaka Insight Meditation*, trans. B. Alan Wallace (Ithaca, N.Y.: Snow Lion, 2002); Thupten Jinpa, *Self, Reality and Reason in Tibetan Philosophy: Tsongkhapa's Quest for the Middle Way* (London: Routledge-Curzon, 2002).

4. *Saṃyutta Nikāya* I:135; *Milindapañhā*, 25.

5. *Saṃyutta Nikāya* I:14; *Itivuttaka* 53.

6. *Sutta Nipāta* 937; *Majjhima Nikāya* III:31.

7. *Saṃyutta Nikāya* II:19; *Saṃyutta Nikāya* II:22; cf. Jay L. Garfield, trans., *The Fundamental Wisdom of the Middle Way: Nāgārjuna's Mūlamadhyamakakārikā* (New York: Oxford University Press, 1995), I, XVII.

8. B. Alan Wallace, *Buddhism with an Attitude: The Tibetan Seven-Point Mind-Training* (Ithaca, N.Y.: Snow Lion, 2001).

9. *Upasīvamāṇavapucchā* of the *Pārāyana*, VI:1069–1076; Luis O. Gomez, "Proto-Mādhyamika in the Pāli Canon," *Philosophy East and West* 26, no. 2 (April 1976): 137–65.

10. *Vajracchedikā Prajñāpāramitā Sūtra;* http://www.plumvillage.org/DharmaDoors/Sutras/chantingbook/Diamond_Sutra.htm.

11. *Vajracchedikā Prajñāpāramitā Sūtra*, 32.

12. Dudjom Rinpoche, *The Illumination of Primordial Wisdom: An Instruction Manual on the Utterly Pure Stage of Perfection of The Powerful and Ferocious Dorje Drolö, Subduer of Demons*, in Gyatrul Rinpoche, *Meditation, Transformation, and Dream Yoga*, trans. B. Alan Wallace and Sangye Khandro (Ithaca, N.Y.: Snow Lion, 2002), 136.

13. Ibid., 136–37.

14. Karma Chagmé, *A Spacious Path to Freedom: Practical Instructions on the Union of Mahāmudrā and Atiyoga*, commentary by Gyatrul Rinpoche, trans. B. Alan Wallace (Ithaca, N.Y.: Snow Lion, 1998), 91–92.

15. Düdjom Lingpa, *The Vajra Essence: From the Matrix of Pure Appearances and Primordial Consciousness, a Tantra on the Self-Originating Nature of Existence*, trans. B. Alan Wallace (Alameda, Calif.: Mirror of Wisdom, 2004), 18–19.

16. Ibid., 44.

19. PRACTICE: THE EMPTINESS OF MATTER

1. Düdjom Lingpa, *The Vajra Essence: From the Matrix of Pure Appearances and Primordial Consciousness, a Tantra on the Self-Originating Nature of Existence*, trans. B. Alan Wallace (Alameda, Calif.: Mirror of Wisdom, 2004), 41–46.

20. THEORY: THE PARTICIPATORY WORLDS OF PHILOSOPHY AND SCIENCE

1. Hilary Putnam, *Realism with a Human Face,* ed. James Conant (Cambridge, Mass.: Harvard University Press, 1990), 30.

2. Charles Taylor, *Sources of the Self: The Making of the Modern Identity* (Cambridge, Mass.: Harvard University Press, 1989), 33–34.

3. George Berkeley, *Three Dialogues Between Hylas and Philonous,* ed. Colin M. Turbayne (1713; reprint, London: Macmillan, 1988).

4. Anālayo Bhikkhu, *Satipaṭṭhāna: The Direct Path to Realization* (Birmingham: Windhorse, 2006), 44–45; *Majjhima Nikāya* II:211; *Saṃyutta Nikāya* IV:139.

5. Immanuel Kant, *Metaphysical Foundations of Natural Science,* trans. James Ellington (1786; reprint, Indianapolis: Bobbs-Merrill, 1970), 8.

6. William James, *Essays in Radical Empiricism* (1912; reprint, New York, Longmans, Green, 1947).

7. B. Alan Wallace, *Hidden Dimensions: The Unification of Physics and Consciousness* (New York: Columbia University Press, 2007), 50–69.

8. Bas C. van Fraassen, "The World of Empiricism," in *Physics and Our View of the World,* ed. Jan Hilgevoort (New York: Cambridge University Press, 1994), 114–34; http://webware .princeton.edu/vanfraas/mss/World92.htm.

9. Taylor, *Sources of the Self,* 33–34.

10. Taylor, *Sources of the Self,* 213.

11. Taylor, *Sources of the Self,* 18.

12. Taylor, *Sources of the Self,* 21.

13. Hilary Putnam, "The Chosen People"; http://bostonreview.net/BR29.1/putnam.html.

14. Hilary Putnam, *Mind, Language and Reality* (Cambridge: Cambridge University Press, 1975), 295–97.

15. Putnam, *Realism with a Human Face,* 28.

16. *Dīgha Nikāya* I:12–29; Anālayo Bhikkhu, *Satipaṭṭhāna,* 45.

17. John Polkinghorne, *Exploring Reality: The Intertwining of Science and Religion* (New Haven: Yale University Press, 2005).

18. Albert Einstein, "Autobiographical Notes," in ref. 27, In *Albert Einstein: Philosopher-Scientist,* ed. P. A. Schlipp (Evanston, Ill.: Library of Living Philosophers, 1949), 81.

19. Wallace, *Hidden Dimensions,* 16–26.

20. Paul C. W. Davies, "An Overview of the Contributions of John Archibald Wheeler," in *Science and Ultimate Reality: Quantum Theory, Cosmology and Complexity, Honoring John Wheeler's 90th Birthday,* ed. John D. Barrow, Paul C. W. Davies, and Charles L. Harper Jr. (Cambridge: Cambridge University Press, 2004), 7.

21. Henning Genz, *Nothingness: The Science of Empty Space* (Cambridge, Mass.: Perseus, 1999), 312.

22. Ibid., 26.

23. Časlav Brukner and Anton Zeilinger, "Information and Fundamental Elements of the Structure of Quantum Theory," in *Time, Quantum and Information*, ed. Lutz Castell and Otfried Ischebeck (Berlin: Springer Verlag, 2003), 352.

24. Anton Zeilinger, "Why the Quantum? 'It' from 'Bit'? A Participatory Universe? Three Far-Reaching Challenges from John Archibald Wheeler and Their Relation to Experiment," in *Science and Ultimate Reality: Quantum Theory, Cosmology and Complexity, Honoring John Wheeler's 90th Birthday*, ed. John D. Barrow, Paul C. W. Davies, and Charles L. Harper Jr. (Cambridge: Cambridge University Press, 2004), 218–19; cf. Carl Friedrich von Weizsäcker, *The Unity of Nature*, trans. Francis J. Zucker (New York: Farrar, Straus & Giroux, 1980), 406.

25. B. Alan Wallace, *Choosing Reality: A Buddhist View of Physics and the Mind* (Ithaca, N.Y.: Snow Lion, 1996); Wallace, *Hidden Dimensions*, ch. 7; L. Q. English, "On the 'Emptiness' of Particles in Condensed-Matter Physics," in *Foundations of Science* 12 (September 29, 2006):155–71; Christian Thomas Kohl, "Buddhism and Quantum Physics: A Strange Parallel of Two Concepts of Reality," *Contemporary Buddhism* 8, no. 1 (May 2007): 69–82; http://ctkohl.googlepages.com.

26. Lisa Randall, *Warped Passages: Unraveling the Mysteries of the Universe's Hidden Dimensions* (New York: Harper Perennial, 2006).

27. Davies, "An Overview of the Contributions of John Archibald Wheeler," 8, 22; Bruce Rosenblum and Fred Kuttner, *Quantum Enigma: Physics Encounters Consciousness* (New York: Oxford University Press, 2006); Henry Stapp, *Mindful Universe: Quantum Mechanics and the Participating Observer* (Berlin: Springer, 2007); Harald Atmanspacher, "Quantum Approaches to Consciousness," in *The Stanford Encyclopedia of Philosophy*, ed. Edward N. Zalta (Stanford: Stanford University Press, 2004); http://plato.stanford .edu/archives/win2004/entries/qt-consciousness/.

28. Mark Buchanan, "Many Worlds: See Me Here, See Me There," *Nature* 448 (July 5, 2007): 15–17; http://www.nature.com/nature/journal/v448/n7149/full/448015a.html.

29. Stephen W. Hawking and Thomas Hertog, "Populating the Landscape: A Top-Down Approach," *Physical Review* 3, no. 73 (2006): 123527; Martin Bojowald, "Unique or Not Unique?" *Nature* 442 (August 31, 2006): 988–90.

21. PRACTICE: RESTING IN TIMELESS CONSCIOUSNESS

1. Padmasambhava, *Natural Liberation: Padmasambhava's Teachings on the Six Bardos* commentary by Gyatrul Rinpoche, trans. B. Alan Wallace (Boston: Wisdom, 1998), 120–22.

22. THEORY: THE LUMINOUS SPACE OF PRISTINE AWARENESS

1. Genesis 1:26; 1 Corinthians 11:7; 2 Corinthians 4:4; Colossians 1:15.

2. Matthew 7:21.

3. Deuteronomy 11:13; Joshua 22:5; Matthew 22:37; Mark 12:30; Luke 10:26–28.

4. John Burnaby, *Amor Dei: A Study of the Religion of St. Augustine* (1938; reprint, Norwich: Canterbury Press, 1991), 104.

5. Matthew 5:48.

6. Luke 17:20–21.

7. Matthew 16:25–26; Luke 17:33; John 3:3.

8. Galatians 2:19.

9. Martin Laird, *Into the Silent Land: A Guide to the Practice of Christian Contemplation* (New York: Oxford University Press, 2006), 11.

10. Ibid., 93.

11. Matthew 13:31–33.

12. Matthew 13:44–46.

13. John 8:12; John 9:5; John 12:46.

14. Saint John of the Cross, *The Living Flame of Love*, I:26, in *The Collected Works of St. John of the Cross*, trans. K. Kavanaugh and R. Rodriguez (Washington, D.C.: Institute of Carmelite Studies, 1979), 589. Cited in Laird, *Into the Silent Land*, 67–68.

15. Evagrius, *The Praktikos*, in *The Praktikos and Chapters on Prayer*, trans. J. Bamberger (Kalamazoo, Mich.: Cistercian Publications, 1981), chap. 34, 54.

16. Saint Gregory Palamas, "The Declaration of the Holy Mountain in Defense of Those Who Devoutly Practice a Life of Stillness," in *The Philokalia: The Complete Text*, trans. G.E.H. Palmer, Philip Sherrard, and Kallistos Ware (London: Faber and Faber, 1995), IV:421, 423–24.

17. Ibid., 251.

18. Nicholas of Cusa, *On Seeking God* (*De quaerendo Deum*, 1445), in *Nicholas of Cusa: Selected Spiritual Writings*, trans. H. Lawrence Bond (New York: Paulist Press, 1997), 225.

19. Nicholas of Cusa, *On the Vision of God* (*De visione Dei*, 1453), in *Nicholas of Cusa: Selected Spiritual Writings*, trans. H. Lawrence Bond (New York: Paulist Press, 1997), 252.

20. Nicholas of Cusa, *On Seeking God*, 231.

21. Ibid., 229.

22. *Aṅguttara Nikāya* I:8–11.

23. *Saṃyutta Nikāya* V:92–93; *Aṅguttara Nikāya* I:61, I:253–55.

24. *Manorathapūraṇī* I:60 (commentary to the *Aṅguttara Nikāya*) and *Atthasālinī* 140 (commentary to the *Dhammasaṅgaṇī*) identify the luminous mind with the *bhavaṅga*.

25. *The Milindapañhā: Being Dialogues Between King Milinda and the Buddhist Sage Nāgasena*, ed. V. Trenckner (Oxford: Pali Text Society, 1997), 299–300; *Milinda's Questions*, trans. I. B. Horner (London: Luzac, 1969).

26. *Dīgha Nikāya* I:223; *Udāna* 80.

27. *Saṃyutta-Nikāya* I:122, II:103, III:53–54, III:124.

28. *The Dhammapada*, ed. Nikunja Vihari Banerjee (New Delhi: Munshiram Manoharlal Publishers, 1989), 39, 267, 412; *Sutta Nipāta* 547, 790, 900.

29. *Saṃyutta-Nikāya* III:54.

30. *Udāna* 8.3.

31. *Aṣṭasāhasrikā Perfection of Wisdom Sūtra*; Peter Harvey, *The Selfless Mind: Personality, Consciousness and Nirvana in Early Buddhism* (Surrey: Curzon Press, 1995), 175.

32. *Anūnatva-apūrnatva-nirdeśa*; http://www.webspawner.com/users/tathagatagarbha11b/index.html.

33. Śāntideva, *A Guide to the Bodhisattva Way of Life*, trans. Vesna A. Wallace and B. Alan Wallace (Ithaca, N.Y.: Snow Lion, 1997), X:55.

34. Thich Nhat Hanh, *Living Buddha, Living Christ* (New York: Riverhead, 1997); H. H. the Dalai Lama, *The Good Heart: A Buddhist Perspective on the Teachings of Jesus*, trans. Geshe Thupten Jinpa (Boston: Wisdom, 1996).

35. *Aṅgulimāla Sūtra*, trans. Stephen Hodge; http://www.webspawner.com/users/tathagatagarbha16/index.html.

36. D. M. Paul, *The Buddhist Feminine Ideal—Queen Śrīmāla and the Tathāgata-garbha* (Missoula, Mont.: Scholar's Press, 1980), ch. 13.

37. *The Dhammapada*, I:1.

38. *Aṅgulimāla Sūtra*.

39. *Laṅkāvatāra Sūtra*, 220; Harvey, *The Selfless Mind*, 176.

40. *Ratnagotra-vibhāga*, vs. 47.

41. *Mahāyāna Mahāparinirvāṇasūtra*, trans. Kosho Yamamoto, rev. Tony Page (London: Nirvana Publications, 1999–2000), ch . 12; *Anūnatva-apūrnatva-nirdeśa*.

42. H. H. the Dalai Lama, *Dzogchen: The Heart Essence of the Great Perfection*, trans. Geshe Thupten Jinpa and Richard Barron (Ithaca, N.Y.: Snow Lion, 2000).

43. Erik Pema Kunsang, trans., *Wellsprings of the Great Perfection: The Lives and Insights of the Early Masters* (Boudhanath, Nepal: Rangjung Yeshe Publications, 2006).

44. Düdjom Lingpa, *The Vajra Essence: From the Matrix of Pure Appearances and Primordial Consciousness, a Tantra on the Self-Originating Nature of Existence*, trans. B. Alan Wallace (Alameda, Calif.: Mirror of Wisdom, 2004), 251.

45. Padmasambhava, *Natural Liberation: Padmasambhava's Teachings on the Six Bardos*, commentary by Gyatrul Rinpoche, trans. B. Alan Wallace (Boston: Wisdom, 1998), 62.

46. H. H. the Dalai Lama, *Dzogchen*, 48–49.

47. Düdjom Lingpa, *The Vajra Essence*, 255.

48. Düdjom Lingpa, *The Vajra Essence*, 244–45.

49. Düdjom Lingpa, *The Vajra Essence*, 251–52.

50. Düdjom Lingpa, *The Vajra Essence*, 115–17.

51. Düdjom Lingpa, *The Vajra Essence*, 321–22.

52. Tulku Urgyen Rinpoche, *Blazing Splendor: The Memoirs of Tulku Urgyen Rinpoche* (Berkeley, Calif.: North Atlantic Books, 2005).

53. Mark 16:9–20; Matthew 28:8–20; Luke 24:7–53.

54. Gail B. Holland, "The Rainbow Body," *IONS: Noetic Sciences Review* 59 (March–May 2002): 33.

55. Ibid., 34.

23. PRACTICE: MEDITATION IN ACTION

1. Düdjom Lingpa, *The Vajra Essence: From the Matrix of Pure Appearances and Primordial Consciousness, a Tantra on the Self-Originating Nature of Existence*, trans. B. Alan Wallace (Alameda, Calif.: Mirror of Wisdom, 2004), 220–27.

24. THEORY: THE UNIVERSE AS A WHOLE

1. Andrei Linde, "Inflation, Quantum Cosmology and the Anthropic Principle," in *Science and Ultimate Reality: Quantum Theory, Cosmology and Complexity, Honoring John Wheeler's 90th Birthday*, ed. John D. Barrow, Paul C. W. Davies, and Charles L. Harper Jr. (Cambridge: Cambridge University Press, 2004), 450–51.
2. Ibid., 451.
3. Paul Davies, *About Time: Einstein's Unfinished Revolution* (New York: Simon & Schuster, 1995); Paul Davies, "That Mysterious Flow," *Scientific American* 16, no. 1 (2006): 6–11.
4. Andre Linde, "Choose Your Own Universe," in *Spiritual Information: 100 Perspectives on Science and Religion*, ed. Charles L. Harper Jr. (West Conshohocken, Penn.: Templeton Foundation Press 2005), 139.
5. Jim Holt, "Where Protons Will Play," *New York Times*, January 14, 2007.
6. Franklin Merrell-Wolff, *Franklin Merrell-Wolff's Experience and Philosophy* (Albany: State University of New York Press, 2003), 284.
7. Daniel C. Matt, "Kabbalah and Contemporary Cosmology: Discovering the Resonances," in *Science, Religion, and the Human Experience*, ed. James Proctor (New York: Oxford University Press, 2005), 129–42.
8. Nicholas of Cusa, *On Seeking God* (*De quaerendo Deum*, 1445) in *Nicholas of Cusa: Selected Spiritual Writings*, trans. H. Lawrence Bond (New York: Paulist Press, 1997), 223.
9. Nicholas of Cusa, *On the Vision of God* (*De visione Dei*, 1453) in *Nicholas of Cusa: Selected Spiritual Writings*, trans. H. Lawrence Bond (New York: Paulist Press, 1997), 261.
10. Karl H. Potter, ed., *Encyclopedia of Indian Philosophies: Advaita Vedānta up to Śaṃkara and His Pupils* (Delhi: Motilal Banarsidass, 1981), 81–87.
11. Düdjom Lingpa, *The Vajra Essence: From the Matrix of Pure Appearances and Primordial Consciousness, a Tantra on the Self-Originating Nature of Existence*, trans. B. Alan Wallace (Alameda, Calif.: Mirror of Wisdom, 2004), 80–87; B. Alan Wallace, *Contemplative Science: Where Buddhism and Neuroscience Converge* (New York: Columbia University Press, 2007), 101–104.

BIBLIOGRAPHY

Amma, T. A. Sarasvati. *Geometry in Ancient and Medieval India*. Delhi: Motilal Banarsidass, 1979.

Anālayo Bhikkhu. *Satipaṭṭhāna: The Direct Path to Realization*. Birmingham, England: Windhorse, 2006.

Asaṅga. *Abhidharmasamuccaya*. Ed. Pralhad Pradhan. Santiniketan: Visva-Bharati, 1950.

Atmanspacher, Harald. "Quantum Approaches to Consciousness." In *The Stanford Encyclopedia of Philosophy*, ed. Edward N. Zalta. Stanford: Stanford University Press, 2004; http://plato.stanford.edu/archives/win2004/entries/qt-consciousness/.

Atmanspacher, Harald and Hans Primas. "The Hidden Side of Wolfgang Pauli." *Journal of Consciousness Studies* 3 (1996): 112–26.

Saint Augustine. *The Free Choice of the Will* (391). Trans. Francis E. Tourscher. Philadelphia: Peter Reilly Co., 1937.

———. *The Literal Meaning of Genesis*. Trans. John Hammond Taylor. New York: Newman Press, 1982.

Banerjee, Nikunja Vihari, ed. *The Dhammapada*. New Delhi: Munshiram Manoharlal Publishers, 1989.

Bareau, A. *Les Sectes Bouddhiques du Petit Véhicule*. Paris: EFEO, 1955.

Barham, Denise. "The Last 48 Hours of Life: A Case Study of Symptom Control for a Patient Taking a Buddhist Approach to Dying." *International Journal of Palliative Nursing* 9, no. 6 (June 2003): 245.

Baruss, Imants. *Science as Spiritual Practice*. Charlottesville, Va.: Imprint Academic, 2007.

Begley, Sharon. "Know Thyself—Man, Rat or Bot." *Newsweek*, April 23, 2007; http://www.news-week.com/id/35401.

———. *Train Your Mind, Change Your Brain: How a New Science Reveals Our Extraordinary Potential to Transform Ourselves*. New York: Ballantine, 2007.

Benson, Herbert. *The Relaxation Response*. New York: Avon, 1976.

Berkeley, George. *Three Dialogues Between Hylas and Philonous* (1713). Ed. Colin M. Turbayne. London: Macmillan, 1988.

Bishop, Scott R. "What Do We Really Know About Mindfulness-Based Stress Reduction?" *Psychosomatic Medicine* 64 (2002): 71–84.

Bishop, Scott R., et al. "Mindfulness: A Proposed Operational Definition." *Clinical Psychology: Science and Practice* 11, no. 3 (Fall 2004): 230–41.

Bitbol, Michel. "Materialism, Stances, and Open-Mindedness." In *Images of Empiricism: Essays on Science and Stances, with a Reply from Bas van Fraassen*, ed. Bradley Monton. Oxford: Oxford University Press, 2007.

Blum, Deborah. *Ghost Hunters: William James and the Search for Scientific Proof of Life After Death*. New York: Penguin, 2006.

Bogart, G. "The Use of Meditation in Psychotherapy: A Review of the Literature." *American Journal of Psychotherapy* 45, no. 3 (July 1991): 383–412.

Bojowald, Martin. "Unique or Not Unique?" *Nature* 442 (August 31, 2006): 988–90.

Bonadonna, R. "Meditation's Impact on Chronic Illness." *Holistic Nursing Practice* 17, no. 6 (November–December 2003): 309–19.

Bruce, Anne and Betty Davies. "Mindfulness in Hospice Care: Practicing Meditation-in-Action." *Qualitative Health Research* 15, no. 10 (2005): 1329–1344.

Brukner, Časlav and Anton Zeilinger. "Information and Fundamental Elements of the Structure of Quantum Theory." In *Time, Quantum and Information*, ed. Lutz Castell and Otfried Ischebeck. Berlin: Springer Verlag, 2003, 323–55.

Buber, Martin. *Between Man and Man*. Trans. Ronald Gregor Smith. New York: Macmillan, 1948.

Buchanan, Mark. "Many Worlds: See Me Here, See Me There." *Nature* 448 (July 5, 2007): 15–17; http://www.nature.com/nature/journal/v448/n7149/full/448015a.html.

Buckelmüller, J., H. P. Landolt, H. H. Stassen, and P. Achermann. "Trait-like Individual Differences in the Human Sleep Electroencephalogram." *Neuroscience* 138 (2006): 351–56.

Buddhadāsa Bhikkhu. *Mindfulness with Breathing: A Manual for Serious Beginners*. Trans. Santikaro Bhikkhu. Boston: Wisdom, 1996.

Buddhaghosa. *The Path of Purification* Trans. Ñāṇamoli Bhikkhu. Kandy, Sri Lanka: Buddhist Publication Society, 1979.

Burnaby, John. *Amor Dei: A Study of the Religion of St. Augustine*. 1938; reprint, Norwich, England: Canterbury Press, 1991.

Chariton of Valamo, Igumen. *The Art of Prayer*. Trans. E. Kadloubovsky and E. Palmer. London: Faber and Faber, 1966.

Churchland, Patricia and Terence J. Sejenowski. "Neural Representation and Neural Computation." In *Mind and Cognition: A Reader*, ed. William G. Lycan. Oxford: Blackwell, 1990, 224–52.

Clément, Olivier. *The Roots of Christian Mysticism*. Trans. T. Berkeley. London: New City Press, 1993.

Cox, Collett. "Mindfulness and Memory: The Scope of *Smṛti* from Early Buddhism to the Sarvāstivādin Abhidharma." In *In the Mirror or Memory: Reflections on Mindfulness and Remembrance in Indian and Tibetan Buddhism*, ed. Janet Gyatso. Albany: State University of New York Press, 1992.

Dahlberg, Carrie Peyton. "Meditation Study Aims to Leap Over Mental Barriers." *Sacramento Bee*, November 29, 2004; http://www.sacbee.com/content/news/story/11608921p-12498535c.html.

H. H. the Dalai Lama. *Freedom in Exile: The Autobiography of the Dalai Lama*. New York: HarperCollins, 1990.

——. *The Good Heart: A Buddhist Perspective on the Teachings of Jesus*. Trans. Geshe Thupten Jinpa. Boston: Wisdom, 1996.

——. *Dzogchen: The Heart Essence of the Great Perfection*. Trans. Geshe Thupten Jinpa and Richard Barron. Ithaca, N.Y.: Snow Lion, 2000.

——. *The Universe in a Single Atom: The Convergence of Science and Spirituality*. New York: Morgan Road, 2005.

H. H. the Dalai Lama and Alex Berzin. *The Gelug/Kagyü Tradition of Mahamudra*. Ithaca, N.Y.: Snow Lion, 1997.

H. H. the Dalai Lama, Dzong-ka-ba, and Jeffrey Hopkins. *Yoga Tantra: Paths to Magical Feats*. Ithaca, N.Y.: Snow Lion, 2005.

Damasio, Antonio. *The Feeling of What Happens: Body and Emotion in the Making of Consciousness*. New York: Harcourt, 1999.

Danziger, Kurt. "The History of Introspection Reconsidered." *Journal of the History of the Behavioral Sciences* 16 (1980): 241–62.

Davidson, Richard J., et al. "Alterations in Brain and Immune Function Produced by Mindfulness Meditation." *Psychosomatic Medicine* 65, no. 4 (July–August 2003): 564–70.

Davies, Bruce A. "Mindfulness in Hospice Care: Practicing Meditation-in-Action." *Qualitative Health Research* 15, no. 10 (December 2005): 1329–1344.

Davies, Paul C. W. *About Time: Einstein's Unfinished Revolution*. New York: Simon & Schuster, 1995.

——. "An Overview of the Contributions of John Archibald Wheeler." In *Science and Ultimate Reality: Quantum Theory, Cosmology and Complexity, Honoring John Wheeler's 90th Birthday*, ed. John D. Barrow, Paul C. W. Davies, and Charles L. Harper Jr. Cambridge: Cambridge University Press, 2004, 3–26.

——. "That Mysterious Flow." *Scientific American* 16, no. 1 (2006): 6–11.

De Gennaro, L., M. Ferrara, F. Vecchio, G. Curcio, and M. Bertini. "An Electroencephalographic Fingerprint of Human Sleep." *NeuroImage* 26 (2005): 114–22.

Dennett, Daniel C. *Content and Consciousness*. New York: Routledge & Kegan Paul, 1969.

——. *Consciousness Explained*. Boston: Little, Brown, 1991.

——. "The Fantasy of First-Person Science" (a written version of a debate with David Chalmers, held at Northwestern University, Evanston, Ill.,. February 15, 2001, supplemented by an e-mail debate with Alvin Goldman); Third Draft. March 1, 2001; http://ase.tufts.edu/cogstud/papers/chalmersdeb3dft.htm.

———. *Breaking the Spell: Religion as a Natural Phenomenon.* New York: Viking, 2006.

Descartes, René. *A Discourse on Method; Meditations on the First Philosophy; Principles of Philosophy.* Trans. John Veitch. London: Everyman, 1994.

———. *Discourse on the Method of Rightly Conducting One's Reason and Seeking the Truth in the Sciences.* Trans. Ian Maclean. New York: Oxford University Press, 2006.

Düdjom Lingpa. *The Vajra Essence: From the Matrix of Pure Appearances and Primordial Consciousness, a Tantra on the Self-Originating Nature of Existence.* Trans. B. Alan Wallace. Alameda, Calif.: Mirror of Wisdom, 2004.

Dudjom Rinpoche. *The Illumination of Primordial Wisdom: An Instruction Manual on the Utterly Pure Stage of Perfection of The Powerful and Ferocious Dorje Drolö, Subduer of Demons.* In Gyatrul Rinpoche, *Meditation, Transformation, and Dream Yoga,* trans. B. Alan Wallace and Sangye Khandro. Ithaca, N.Y.: Snow Lion, 2002, 133–42.

Einstein, Albert. "Autobiographical Notes." In *Albert Einstein: Philosopher-Scientist,* ed. P. A. Schlipp. Evanston, Ill.: Library of Living Philosophers, 1949, 2–95.

Ekman, Paul. *Emotions Revealed: Recognizing Faces and Feelings to Improve Communication and Emotional Life.* New York: Times Books, 2003.

Ekman, Paul, Richard J. Davidson, Matthieu Ricard, and B. Alan Wallace. "Buddhist and Psychological Perspectives on Emotions and Well-Being." *Current Directions in Psychology* 14, no. 2 (2005): 59–63.

Ellison, Katherine. "Mastering Your Own Mind." *Psychology Today* (October 2006); http://www.psychologytoday.com/ and click on "Mastering Your Own Mind."

English, L. Q. "On the 'Emptiness' of Particles in Condensed-Matter Physics." *Foundations of Science* 12 (September 29, 2006): 155–71.

Epstein, Mark. *Thoughts Without a Thinker: Psychotherapy from a Buddhist Perspective.* New York: Basic Books, 1995.

Evagrius. *The Praktikos.* In *The Praktikos and Chapters on Prayer,* trans. J. Bamberger. Kalamazoo, Mich: Cistercian Publications, 1981.

Feynman, Richard P. *The Character of Physical Law.* Cambridge, Mass.: MIT Press, 1965.

Finelli, L. A., P. Achermann, and A. Borbély. "Individual Fingerprints in Human Sleep EEG Topography." *Neuropsychopharmacology* 25 (2001): S57–S62.

Finkelstein, David. "Ur Theory and Space-Time Structure." In *Time, Quantum and Information,* ed. Lutz Castell and Otfried Ischebeck. Berlin: Springer Verlag, 2003, 399–409.

Foote, Allison L. and Jonathan D. Crystal. "Metacognition in the Rat." *Current Biology* 17 (March 20, 2007): 551–55.

Freud, Sigmund. *Civilization and Its Discontents.* Trans. and ed. James Strachey. New York: Norton, 1961.

Garfield, Jay L., trans. *The Fundamental Wisdom of the Middle Way: Nāgārjuna's Mūlamadhyamakakārikā.* New York: Oxford University Press, 1995.

Gedün Lodrö, Geshe. *Walking Through Walls: A Presentation of Tibetan Meditation.* Trans. and ed. Jeffrey Hopkins. Ithaca, N.Y.: Snow Lion, 1992.

Genz, Henning. *Nothingness: The Science of Empty Space.* Cambridge, Mass.: Perseus, 1999.

Gethin, Rupert M. L. *The Buddhist Path to Awakening.* Oxford: Oneworld, 2001.

Goleman, Daniel, ed. *Healing Emotions: Conversations with the Dalai Lama on Mindfulness, Emotions, and Health.* Boston: Shambhala, 1997.

——. *Destructive Emotions: A Scientific Dialogue with the Dalai Lama.* New York: Bantam Doubleday, 2002.

Gomez, Luis O. "Proto-Mādhyamika in the Pāli Canon." *Philosophy East and West* 26, no. 2 (April 1976): 137–65.

——. *The Land of Bliss: The Paradise of the Buddha of Measureless Light.* Honolulu: University of Hawai'i Press, 1996.

Gupta, Bina. *The Disinterested Witness: A Fragment of Advaita Vedānta Phenomenology.* Evanston, Ill.: Northwestern University Press, 1998.

Harvey, Peter. "The Mind-Body Relationship in Pāli Buddhism—a Philosophical Investigation." *Asian Philosophy* 3, no. 1 (1993): 29–41.

——. *The Selfless Mind: Personality, Consciousness and Nirvana in Early Buddhism.* Surrey: Curzon Press, 1995.

Hawking, Stephen W. and Thomas Hertog. "Populating the Landscape: A Top-Down Approach." *Physical Review* 3, no. 73 (2006): 123527.

Henig, Robin Marantz. "The Real Transformers." *New York Times,* July 29, 2007; http://www.nytimes.com/2007/07/29/magazine/29robots-t.html?_r=1&adxnnl=1&oref=slogin&adxnnlx=1185711249-XL9nqJdFDjGpK4ck3uvoxQ.

Hilgevoort, Jan., ed. *Physics and Our View of the World.* New York: Cambridge University Press, 1994.

Holland, Gail Bernice. "The Rainbow Body." *IONS: Noetic Sciences Review* 59 (March–May 2002): 32–35.

Holmes, K. H. and K. Holmes, trans. *The Changeless Continuity.* 2nd ed. Eskdalemuir, Scotland: Karma Drubgyud Darjay Ling, 1985.

Holt, Jim. "Where Protons Will Play." *New York Times,* January 14, 2007.

Horner, I. B., trans. *Milinda's Questions.* London: Luzac, 1969.

James, William. *The Principles of Psychology.* 1890; reprint, New York: Dover, 1950.

——. "A Plea for Psychology as a Science." *Philosophical Review* 1 (1892): 146–53.

——. "Does Consciousness Exist?" (1905). In *The Writings of William James,* ed. John J. McDermott. Chicago: University of Chicago Press, 1977, 169–83.

——. *Some Problems of Philosophy: A Beginning of an Introduction to Philosophy.* London: Longmans, Green, 1911.

——. *Essays in Radical Empiricism.* 1912; reprint, New York: Longmans, Green, 1947.

——. *Essays in Religion and Morality.* Cambridge, Mass.: Harvard University Press, 1989.

Jamgön Kongtrul Lodrö Tayé. *Myriad Worlds: Buddhist Cosmology in Abhidharma, Kālacakra and Dzog-chen.* Trans. and ed. the International Translation Committee. Ithaca, N.Y.: Snow Lion, 1995.

Jha, Amishi P., Jason Krompinger, and Michael J. Baime. "Mindfulness Training Modifies Subsystems of Attention. *Cognitive, Affective, and Behavioral Neuroscience* 7, no. 2 (2007): 109–19.

Jiang, Tao. *Yogācāra Buddhism and Modern Psychology on the Subliminal Mind.* Society for Asian and Comparative Philosophy Monographs, No. 21. Honolulu: University of Hawai'i Press, 2006.

Jinpa, Thupten. *Self, Reality and Reason in Tibetan Philosophy: Tsongkhapa's Quest for the Middle Way.* London: RoutledgeCurzon, 2002.

Saint John of the Cross. "The Living Flame of Love," I:26. In *The Collected Works of St. John of the Cross,* trans. K. Kavanaugh and R. Rodriguez. Washington, D.C.: Institute of Carmelite Studies, 1979.

Kandel, Eric R. *In Search of Memory: The Emergence of a New Science of Mind.* New York: Norton, 2007.

Kant, Immanuel. *Metaphysical Foundations of Natural Science* (1786). Trans. James Ellington. Indianapolis: Bobbs-Merrill, 1970.

Karma Chagmé. *A Spacious Path to Freedom: Practical Instructions on the Union of Mahāmudrā and Atiyoga.* Commentary by Gyatrul Rinpoche Trans. B. Alan Wallace. Ithaca, N.Y.: Snow Lion, 1998.

Karma Thinley. *History of 16 Karmapas.* Boston: Shambhala, 2001.

Keating, Thomas. *Open Mind, Open Heart: The Contemplative Dimension of the Gospel.* New York: Crossroad, 2001.

Kelly, Edward F., Emily Williams Kelly, Adam Crabtree, Alan Gauld, Michael Grosso, and Bruce Greyson. *Irreducible Mind: Toward a Psychology for the 21st Century.* Lanham, Md.: Rowman & Littlefield, 2007.

Koch, Christof. *The Quest for Consciousness: A Neurobiological Approach.* Englewood, Colo.: Roberts, 2004.

Kohl, Christian Thomas. "Buddhism and Quantum Physics: A Strange Parallel of Two Concepts of Reality." *Contemporary Buddhism* 8, no. 1 (May 2007): 69–82.

Kunsang, Erik Pema, trans. *Wellsprings of the Great Perfection: The Lives and Insights of the Early Masters.* Boudhanath, Nepal: Rangjung Yeshe Publications, 2006.

LaBerge, Stephen. "Lucid Dreaming and the Yoga of the Dream State: A Psychophysiological Perspective." In *Buddhism and Science: Breaking New Ground,* ed. B. Alan Wallace. New York: Columbia University Press, 2003, 233–58.

LaBerge, Stephen and Howard Rheingold. *Exploring the World of Lucid Dreaming.* New York: Ballantine, 1990.

Laird, Martin. *Into the Silent Land: A Guide to the Practice of Christian Contemplation.* New York: Oxford University Press, 2006.

Lamme, Victor A. F. "Towards a True Neural Stance on Consciousness." *TRENDS in Cognitive Sciences* 10, no. 11 (November 2006): 494–501.

Lamrimpa, Gen. *Realizing Emptiness: Madhyamaka Insight Meditation.* Trans. B. Alan Wallace. Ithaca, N.Y.: Snow Lion, 2002.

Lau, Hakwan C., Robert D. Rogers, and Richard E. Passingham. "Manipulating the Experienced Onset of Intention After Action Execution." *Journal of Cognitive Neuroscience* 19, no. 1 (January 2007): 81–90.

Lazar, Sara. W., C. E. Kerr, R. H. Wasserman, J. R. Gray, D. N. Greve, M. T. Treadway, M. McGarvey, B. T. Quinn, J. A. Dusek, H. Benson, S. L. Rauch, C. I. Moore, and B. Fischl. "Meditation Experience Is Associated with Increased Cortical Thickness." *Neuroreport* 16 (2005): 893–97.

Leonard, Ron. *The Transcendent Philosophy of Franklin Merrell-Wolff.* Albany: State University of New York Press, 1999.

Leuchter, Andrew F. et al. "Changes in Brain Function of Depressed Subjects During Treatment with Placebo." *American Journal of Psychiatry* 159 (2002): 122–29.

Linde, Andre. "Inflation, Quantum Cosmology and the Anthropic Principle." In *Science and Ultimate Reality: Quantum Theory, Cosmology and Complexity, Honoring John Wheeler's 90th Birthday,* ed. John D. Barrow, Paul C. W. Davies, and Charles L. Harper Jr. Cambridge: Cambridge University Press, 2004, 426–58.

———. "Choose Your Own Universe." In *Spiritual Information: 100 Perspectives on Science and Religion,* ed. Charles L. Harper Jr. West Conshohocken, Penn.: Templeton Foundation Press, 2005, 137–41.

Lozang Chökyi Gyaltsen, Panchen. *The Great Seal of Voidness.* In *The Mahāmudrā Eliminating the Darkness of Ignorance,* trans. Alex Berzin. Dharamsala: Library of Tibetan Works and Archives, 1978.

Lutz, Antoine et al. "Long-term Meditators Self-Induce High-Amplitude Gamma Synchrony During Mental Practice." *Proceedings of the National Academy of Science* 101, no. 49 (November 16, 2004): 16369–16373.

MacLean, C. R., et al. "Effects of the Transcendental Meditation Program on Adaptive Mechanisms: Changes in Hormone Levels and Responses to Stress After Four Months of Practice." *Psychoneuroendocrinology* 22, no. 4 (May 1997): 277–95.

McDermott, Charlene. "Yogic Direct Awareness as Means of Valid Cognition in Dharmakīrti and Rgyal-tshab." In *Mahāyāna Meditation: Theory and Practice,* ed. Minoru Kiyota. Honolulu: University of Hawai'i Press, 1978, 144–66.

McDermott, John J., ed. *The Writings of William James.* Chicago: University of Chicago Press, 1977.

Matt, Daniel C. "*Ayin:* The Concept of Nothingness in Jewish Mysticism." In *The Problem of Pure Consciousness: Mysticism and Philosophy,* ed. Robert K. C. Forman. New York: Oxford University Press, 1990.

———. "Kabbalah and Contemporary Cosmology: Discovering the Resonances." In *Science, Religion, and the Human Experience,* ed. James Proctor. New York: Oxford University Press, 2005, 129–42.

Mensky, Michael B. "Concept of Consciousness in the Context of Quantum Mechanics." *Physics—Uspekhi* 48, no. 4 (2005): 389–409.

Merrell-Wolff, Franklin. *Mathematics, Philosophy, and Yoga: A Lecture Series Presented at the Los Olivos Conference Room in Phoenix, Arizona in 1966.* Phoenix, Ariz.: Phoenix Philosophical Press, 1995.

———. *Franklin Merrell-Wolff's Experience and Philosophy.* Albany: State University of New York Press, 2003.

Merton, Thomas. *Cassian and the Fathers: Initiation Into the Monastic Tradition.* Kalamazoo, Mich.: Cistercian Publications, 2005.

Ñāṇamoli, Bhikkhu. *The Life of the Buddha According to the Pali Canon.* Kandy, Sri Lanka: Buddhist Publication Society, 1992.

Ñāṇamoli, Bhikkhu and Bhikkhu Bodhi, trans. *The Middle Length Discourses of the Buddha.* Boston: Wisdom, 1995.

Nauriyal, D. K., ed. *Buddhist Thought and Applied Psychology: Transcending the Boundaries.* London: Routledge-Curzon, 2006.

Nicholas of Cusa. *On Seeking God (De quaerendo Deum, 1445).* In *Nicholas of Cusa: Selected Spiritual Writings,* trans. H. Lawrence Bond. New York: Paulist Press, 1997.

——. *On the Vision of God (De visione Dei, 1453).* In *Nicholas of Cusa: Selected Spiritual Writings,* trans. H. Lawrence Bond. New York: Paulist Press, 1997.

Pa-Auk Tawya Sayadaw. *Knowing and Seeing.* Kuala Lumpur, Malaysia: WAVE Publications, 2003.

Padmasambhava. *Natural Liberation: Padmasambhava's Teachings on the Six Bardos.* Commentary by Gyatrul Rinpoche. Trans. B. Alan Wallace. Boston: Wisdom, 1998.

Palamas, Saint Gregory. "In Defense of Those Who Devoutly Practice a Life of Stillness." In *The Philokalia: The Complete Text,* trans. G.E.H. Palmer, Philip Sherrard, and Kallistos Ware. London: Faber and Faber, 1995, IV:331–42.

——. "The Declaration of the Holy Mountain in Defense of Those Who Devoutly Practice a Life of Stillness." In *The Philokalia: The Complete Text,* trans. G.E.H. Palmer, Philip Sherrard, and Kallistos Ware. London: Faber and Faber, 1995, IV:418–25.

Palmer, G.E.H., Philip Sherrard, and Kallistos Ware, trans. *The Philokalia: The Complete Text,* Vol. IV. London: Faber and Faber, 1995.

Paul, D. M. *The Buddhist Feminine Ideal—Queen Śrīmālā and the Tathāgata-garbha.* Missoula: Montana Scholar's Press, 1980.

Pieper, Josef. *Happiness and Contemplation.* Trans. Richard and Clara Winston. Chicago: Henry Regnery, 1966.

Plato. *The Collected Dialogues of Plato.* Ed. Edith Hamilton and Huntington Cairns. Trans. Hugh Tredennick. Bollingen Series LXXI. Princeton: Princeton University Press, 1961.

——. *The Republic.* Trans. R. E. Allen. New Haven: Yale University Press, 2006.

Polkinghorne, John. *Exploring Reality: The Intertwining of Science and Religion.* New Haven: Yale University Press, 2005.

Potter, Karl H., ed. *Encyclopedia of Indian Philosophies: Advaita Vedānta up to Śaṃkara and His Pupils.* Delhi: Motilal Banarsidass, 1981.

Putnam, Hilary. *Mind, Language and Reality.* Cambridge: Cambridge University Press, 1975.

——. *Realism with a Human Face.* Ed. James Conant. Cambridge, Mass.: Harvard University Press, 1990.

——. "The Chosen People"; http://bostonreview.net/BR29.1/putnam.html.

Rabten, Geshe. *The Mind and Its Functions.* Trans. Stephen Batchelor. Mt. Pèlerin, France: Tharpa Choeling, 1979.

——. *Echoes of Voidness.* Trans. and ed. Stephen Batchelor. London: Wisdom, 1986.

Raju, P. T. *Structural Depths of Indian Thought.* Albany: State University of New York Press, 1985.

Randall, Lisa. *Warped Passages: Unraveling the Mysteries of the Universe's Hidden Dimensions*. New York: Harper Perennial, 2006.

Richards, T. A., et al. "A Qualitative Examination of a Spiritually-Based Intervention and Self-Management in the Workplace." *Nursing Science Quarterly* (July 2006).

Rosenblum, Bruce and Fred Kuttner. *Quantum Enigma: Physics Encounters Consciousness*. New York: Oxford University Press, 2006.

Sahagun, Louis. "The Dalai Lama Has It—but Just What Is 'It'?" *Los Angeles Times*, December 9, 2006, B2.

Śāntideva. *A Guide to the Bodhisattva Way of Life*. Trans. Vesna A. Wallace and B. Alan Wallace. Ithaca, N.Y.: Snow Lion, 1997.

Scholem, Gershom, ed. *Zohar, The Book of Splendor: Basic Readings from the Kabbalah*. New York: Schocken, 1995.

Searle, John R. *Consciousness and Language*. Cambridge: Cambridge University Press, 2002.

——. *Mind: A Brief Introduction*. New York: Oxford University Press, 2004.

Segal, Zindel V., et al. *Mindfulness-Based Cognitive Therapy for Depression: A New Approach to Preventing Relapse*. New York: Guilford, 2002.

——. "Mindfulness-Based Cognitive Therapy: Theoretical Rationale and Empirical Status." In *Mindfulness and Acceptance: Expanding the Cognitive-Behavioral Tradition*, ed. S. C. Hayes, et al. New York: Guilford, 2004.

Seife, Charles. *Decoding the Universe: How the New Science of Information Is Explaining Everything in the Cosmos, from Our Brains to Black Holes*. New York: Viking, 2006.

Shabkar Tsokdrug Rangdröl. *The Flight of the Garuda*. In *The Flight of the Garuda*, trans. Erik Pema Kunsang, 4th ed. Kathmandu: Rangjung Yeshe Publications, 1993, 13–99.

Sharma, Poonam and Jim B. Tucker. "Cases of the Reincarnation Type with Memories from the Intermission Between Lives." *Journal of Near-Death Studies* 23, no. 2 (Winter 2004): 101–18.

Silver, Lee. "Life 2.0." *Newsweek International*, June 4, 2007; http://www.msnbc.msn.com/id/18882828/site/newsweek/.

Skinner, B. F. *Science and Human Behavior*. New York: Macmillan, 1953.

——. "Behaviorism at Fifty." In *Behaviorism and Phenomenology: Contrasting Bases for Modern Psychology*, ed. T. W. Wann. Chicago: University of Chicago Press, 1964, 79–108.

——. *About Behaviorism*. New York: Knopf, 1974.

Sobel, Dava. *Galileo's Daughter: A Historical Memoir of Science, Faith, and Love*. New York: Penguin, 2000.

Soma Thera, trans. *Kalama Sutta: The Buddha's Charter of Free Inquiry*. Kandy, Sri Lanka: Buddhist Publication Society, 1981.

Speca, M., et al. "A Randomized Wait-List Controlled Clinical Trial: The Effect of a Mindfulness Meditation-Based Stress Reduction Program on Mood and Symptoms of Stress in Cancer Outpatients." *Psychosomatic Medicine* 62, no. 5 (September–October 2000): 613–22.

Stapp, Henry. *Mindful Universe: Quantum Mechanics and the Participating Observer*. Berlin: Springer, 2007.

Stevenson, Ian, M.D. *Where Reincarnation and Biology Intersect*. New York: Praeger, 1997.

————. *Reincarnation and Biology: A Contribution to the Etiology of Birthmarks and Birth Defects.* New York: Praeger, 1997.

Sujato, Bhikkhu. *A History of Mindfulness: How Insight Worsted Tranquility in the Satipatthana Sutta.* Taipei: The Corporate Body of the Buddha Educational Foundation, 2005.

Saint Symeon the New Theologian. "The Three Methods of Prayer." In *The Philokalia: The Complete Text,* trans. G.E.H. Palmer, Philip Sherrard, and Kallistos Ware. London: Faber and Faber, 1995, IV:67–75.

Tang, Yi-Yuan, et al. "Short-Term Meditation Training Improves Attention and Self-Regulation." *PNAS Early Edition,* August 16, 2007; www.pnas.org/cgi/doi/10.1073/pnas.0707678104.

Taylor, Charles. *Sources of the Self: The Making of the Modern Identity.* Cambridge, Mass.: Harvard University Press, 1989.

Teasdale, John D., et al. "Prevention of Relapse/Recurrence in Major Depression by Mindfulness-Based Cognitive Therapy." *Journal of Consulting and Clinical Psychology* 68, no. 4 (August 2000): 615–23.

Thackeray, H. St. J., R. Marcus, A. Wikgren, and L. H. Feldman, trans. *Josephus.* Loeb Classical Library. London: Heinemann, 1956.

Thich Nhat Hanh. *Living Buddha, Living Christ.* New York: Riverhead, 1997.

Thompson, Evan. *Mind in Life: Biology, Phenomenology, and the Sciences of Mind.* Cambridge, Mass.: Belknap Press, 2007.

Tinguely, G., L. A. Finelli, H.-P. Landolt, A. A. Borbély, and P. Achermann. "Functional EEG Topography in Sleep and Waking: State-Dependent and State-Independent Features." *NeuroImage* 32 (2006): 283–92.

Trenckner, V., ed. *The Milindapañhā: Being Dialogues Between King Milinda and the Buddhist Sage Nāgasena.* Oxford: Pali Text Society, 1997.

Tucker, Jim. *Life Before Life: A Scientific Investigation of Children's Memories of Previous Lives.* New York: St. Martin's Press, 2005.

Unno, Mark, ed. *Buddhism and Psychotherapy Across Cultures: Essays on Theories and Practices.* Boston: Wisdom, 2006.

Urgyen Rinpoche, Tulku. *Blazing Splendor: The Memoirs of Tulku Urgyen Rinpoche.* Berkeley, Calif.: North Atlantic Books, 2005.

van Fraassen, Bas C. *The Scientific Image.* New York: Oxford University Press, 1980.

————. "From Vicious Circle to Infinite Regress and Back Again." In *Proceedings of the 1992 Biennial Meeting of the Philosophy of Science Association,* ed. D. Hull, M. Forbes, and K. Okruhlick, Vol. 2 1993 (in *Philosophy of Science*).

————. "The World of Empiricism." In *Physics and Our View of the World,* ed. Jan Hilgevoort. New York: Cambridge University Press, 1994, 114–34; http://webware.princeton.edu/vanfraas/mss/World92.htm.

————. *The Empirical Stance.* New Haven: Yale University Press, 2002.

von Weizsäcker, Carl Friedrich. *The Unity of Nature.* Trans. Francis J. Zucker. New York: Farrar, Straus & Giroux, 1980.

Wallace, B. Alan. *Choosing Reality: A Buddhist View of Physics and the Mind.* Ithaca, N.Y.: Snow Lion, 1996.

———. *The Taboo of Subjectivity: Toward a New Science of Consciousness.* New York: Oxford University Press, 2000.

———. *Buddhism with an Attitude: The Tibetan Seven-Point Mind-Training.* Ithaca, N.Y.: Snow Lion, 2001.

———. *Balancing the Mind: A Tibetan Buddhist Approach to Refining Attention.* Ithaca, N.Y.: Snow Lion, 2005.

———. *Genuine Happiness: Meditation as the Path to Fulfillment.* Hoboken, N.J.: Wiley, 2005.

———. "Vacuum States of Consciousness: A Tibetan Buddhist View." In *Buddhist Thought and Applied Psychology: Transcending the Boundaries,* ed. D. K. Nauriyal. London: Routledge-Curzon, 2006, 112–21.

———. *Contemplative Science: Where Buddhism and Neuroscience Converge.* New York: Columbia University Press, 2007.

———. *Hidden Dimensions: The Unification of Physics and Consciousness.* New York: Columbia University Press, 2007.

Wallace, B. Alan, ed. *Buddhism and Science: Breaking New Ground.* New York: Columbia University Press, 2003.

Wallace, B. Alan and Shauna Shapiro. "Mental Balance and Well-Being: Building Bridges Between Buddhism and Western Psychology." *American Psychologist* 161, no. 7 (October 2006): 690–701; http://www.sbinstitute.com/mentalbalance.pdf.

Wallace, B. Alan and Brian Hodel. *Embracing Mind: The Common Ground of Science and Spirituality.* Boston: Shambhala, 2008.

Walshe, Maurice. *The Long Discourses of the Buddha: A Translation of the Dīgha Nikāya.* Somerville, Mass.: Wisdom, 1995.

Ward, Sister Benedicta. *The Sayings of the Desert Fathers: The Alphabetical Collection.* 2nd ed. London: Oxford University Press, 1981.

Wasner, Maria, et al. "Effects of Spiritual Care Training for Palliative Care Professionals." *Palliative Medicine* 19 (2005): 99–104.

Watson, John B. *Behaviorism.* 1913; reprint, New York: Norton, 1970.

———. "Psychology as a Behaviorist Views It." *Psychological Review* 20 (1913): 158–77.

Wegner, Daniel M. *The Illusion of Conscious Will.* Cambridge, Mass.: MIT Press, 2003.

Werner, K. "Indian Concepts of Human Personality in Relation to the Doctrine of the Soul." *Journal of the Royal Asiatic Society* 1 (1988): 73–97.

Wheeler, John Archibald. "Law Without Law." In *Quantum Theory and Measurement,* ed. John Archibald Wheeler and Wojciech Hubert Zurek. Princeton: Princeton University Press, 1983, 182–213.

Wiebe, Phillip H. "Religious Experience, Cognitive Science, and the Future of Religion." In *The Oxford Handbook of Religion and Science,* ed. Philip Clayton and Zachary Simpson. New York: Oxford University Press, 2006, 503–22.

Yamamoto, Kosho, trans. *Mahāyāna Mahāparinirvāṇasūtra.* Tony Page, rev. London: Nirvana, 1999–2000.

Yokoi, Yuho. *Zen Master Dogen: An Introduction with Selected Writings.* New York: Weatherhill, 1976.

Zajonc, Arthur, ed. *The New Physics and Cosmology: Dialogues with the Dalai Lama*. New York: Oxford University Press, 2004.

Zeilinger, Anton. "Why the Quantum? 'It' from 'Bit'? A Participatory Universe? Three Far-Reaching Challenges from John Archibald Wheeler and Their Relation to Experiment." In *Science and Ultimate Reality: Quantum Theory, Cosmology and Complexity, Honoring John Wheeler's 90th Birthday*, ed. John D. Barrow, Paul C. W. Davies, and Charles L. Harper Jr. Cambridge: Cambridge University Press, 2004, 201–20.

INDEX

biology: and human nature, 4; life force hypothesis, 121; Oparin's hypothesis, 121–22; origin of life, 121–22, 128–31; and traditional hierarchy of scientific inquiry, 112. *See also* neuroscience

birthmarks, 107

bliss: and buddha nature, 177; and mindfulness of breathing meditation, 44; and nirvana, 175, 181; and *samadhi*, 12; and substrate consciousness, 91, 93

bodhisattva, 46, 176–77, 192

body: body–mind imbalance, 42–43; and conservation of consciousness, 95–96; at death, 183–85; embodiment following interval between death and rebirth, 101; and emptiness of matter meditation, 151–52; and mantras, 44; and Merrell-Wolff's experiences in transcending physical embodiment, 192; mind-made body, 100; nirvana and freedom from physical embodiment, 173; out-of-body experiences, 110–11; and personal identity, 59, 118, 140–44, 146; rainbow body, 183–85; reincarnation and imprinting from experiences, 107, 116–17; self-healing capacity of, 60; and the soul in Judeo-Christian tradition, 102–3; and tests of reincarnation, 117. *See also* brain; health benefits of meditation; mind–brain relationship; neuroscience; reincarnation; sensory perception

Book of Formation (Kabbalist text), 104

Book of Splendor (Kabbalist text), 104

brain: and conservation of consciousness, 95–96; and emotions, 55; neuroplasticity studies, 27–28; and scientific studies of meditation, 27–36; and substrate, 95–96. *See also* mind–brain relationship; neuroscience

breathing, mindfulness of, 39–40, 42–46

"brightly shining mind," 174–77, 181

Brooks, Rodney, 124

Buber, Martin, 128

Buddha: and bodhisattva way of life, 46; and "brightly shining mind," 174–76; on dependent origination, 144–45; enlightenment of, 43, 104; on experiential spirituality vs. faith-based religion, 12, 125; on the five hindrances, 85; and Four Noble Truths, 13; and the ground state of consciousness, 89; on liberation through one's own efforts, 59; meditation studies, 12; and mindfulness (*sati*), 62; and mindfulness of breathing exercise, 43–44; and the nature of reality, 139–40, 154–55; on necessary conditions for emergence of human psyche, 104, 117–18; on nirvana, 175; on origins of good and evil, joy and sorrow, 56, 140; and reincarnation, 12, 113; and *samadhi*, 80, 83–85; and suffering, 12–13; teachers of, 12

buddha nature, 176–86, 196

Buddhaghosa, 62–64, 84, 114

Buddhism: and causes of suffering, 12–13, 55–56, 142–45, 148; dependent origination, 144–45, 150; and expansion of ideals from individual liberation to liberation of all beings, 46, 176, 177, 181, 192; and karma, 104, 105, 107, 108; meditation in (*see* Buddhist contemplative tradition; meditation); and the nature of reality, 139–50, 162, 179–86, 194–95; parallels with modern physics, 159–60; rainbow body, 183–85; and reincarnation, 101, 104–5, 108–9, 113–15, 117–18; and the soul, 93. *See also* Great Perfection (Dzogchen) school of Tibetan Buddhism; Mahayana Buddhism; Theravada Buddhism; Tibetan Buddhism; Zen Buddhism

Buddhist contemplative tradition: and "brightly shining mind," 174–76; and enlightenment, 176–86; and introspection, 61–65; and inversion of consciousness, 80–89; lifestyle supportive of meditative practice, 64; and mindfulness (*sati*), 62–65; observing the mind, 57–59; orientation of meditation practice, 13, 59; origins of, 11–13;

samadhi, 80, 82–86; stages of meditative stabilization, 84–85. *See also* meditation; *specific contemplatives*

California Pacific Medical Center, 29–30
Cassian, John, 11
causality: and closure principle, 159; and dependent origination, 144–45; and mind-brain relationship, 23–24, 55; and reincarnation, 106
CEB. *See* Cultivating Emotional Balance (CEB) program
chariot metaphor, 144–46
Charvaka, 54
Chetsün Senge Shora, 184
Chetsün Senge Wangchuck, 184
children: memories of intermediate period between death and rebirth, 109–10; past life memories of, 107; training in enhanced attention, 31–32
Christian contemplative tradition, 44–46; and cosmology, 193–94; and death, 83, 85; Desert Fathers, 11, 75, 170; explorations on the nature of consciousness, 75–77, 83; and God, 46; Greek Orthodox contemplative tradition, 44–45, 56, 58–59, 75–76; and meditation on breath, 44–45; and observing the mind, 56–57; orientation of meditation practice, 13, 58–59; possible Greek influences on, 9–10; and reincarnation, 10, 11; Roman Catholic contemplative tradition, 58–59; Russian Orthodox contemplative tradition, 76; and unity with God, 170–72; and watchfulness/discernment, 63, 75. *See also specific contemplatives*
Christianity: and breath of life, 44–46; human nature and good vs. evil, 3–4, 53–56; and kingdom of heaven, 169–74, 176; and reincarnation, 101–4; and rise of modern science, 15–18, 189; and the soul, 102–5, 190. *See also* Bible; Jesus
closure principle, 159

cognitive science: assumptions about future accomplishments of, 130, 158–59; conclusions about consciousness predetermined by limitations of methods of inquiry, 132; lack of sophisticated means for examining mental events, 24–25, 67, 78, 93; and mind-brain relationship, 24, 105–6, 122–23; and traditional hierarchy of scientific inquiry, 112. *See also* neuroscience; psychology
cognizance, as quality of consciousness, 89
consciousness, 75–93; and artificial intelligence, 123–24, 134; awareness of consciousness meditation, 71–73, 78–88; Buddhist "brightly shining mind" dimension of, 174–77, 181; Buddhist inversion of, 80–82; Christian contemplative explorations of, 75–77, 83; conclusions about consciousness predetermined by limitations of methods of inquiry, 132; and contemplative skepticism about scientific approach to, 131–34; and death, 83 (*see also* reincarnation); defining characteristics of, 89–91; ground state of, 89–96; James and, 155; lack of authentic science of consciousness, 77–78 (*see also* skepticism); Merrell-Wolff and, 79–81; and modern physics, 189–91; need for "top down" study of, 165; and philosophy, 77–80, 153–57; principle of conservation of, 95–96; and *samadhi*, 82–86; science's inability to detect, 78, 123–25, 127, 131, 133, 164; scientific definition of, 124–25, 133–34; Shankara and, 79; 20th-century approaches to, 77–80. *See also* brain; enlightenment; identity; mind; mind–brain relationship; nirvana; primordial consciousness; soul; substrate consciousness
contemplative inquiry, scientific, 5, 60; marginalization of, 16, 21–22, 25, 132; need for years of training in, 132; and reincarnation, 113–18
contemplative insight, 5; Christian doctrine decided by church councils rather than

ecosphere, 42

EEG signatures, as test of reincarnation, 117

Einstein, Albert, 78, 158

Ekman, Paul, 33–34

élan vital, 121–22

Elijah, 10, 102

embryo, 104, 118

emergent properties, 23–24, 54, 122–23

emotions: and artificial intelligence, 123–24; and causes of suffering, 55–56, 145; emotional health, 4, 32–35, 42–44, 60–61; and observing the mind, 68; and substrate, 95

empiricism, 150, 153–57

energy: divine energy (Jewish mysticism), 193; energy of primordial consciousness (*jñanavayu*), 179–80, 194; substrate permeated by energy field, 94 (*see also* life force)

enlightenment, 175–86; and rainbow body, 183–85; and the welfare of other sentient beings, 46, 176, 177, 181, 192

Enneads (Plotinus), 10

Epicurus, 54, 55

epigenetics, 28–29

Essenes, 9–10

Evagrius of Pontus, 11, 44, 170

evil, 3–4, 53–56, 177

evolution, Darwinian, 106, 128–30

excitation, as attentional imbalance, 63–64, 84, 177

"extraordinary claims require extraordinary evidence" principle, 128–31

eyes, and meditation practice, 39–40

Feynman, Richard, 135

Four Noble Truths, 13

free will, 15, 20, 53–55

Freud, Sigmund, 4, 21, 54

frozen time problem, 190–91

Galileo Galilei, 16–18, 67, 78, 82, 172, 189

gamma wave activity in the brain, 31

The Gate of Reincarnation (Kabbalist text), 104

Geshe Gedün Lodrö, 114

Geshe Lamrimpa, 185

gnosis, 11

Gnostic philosophy, 11

God: Berkeley on (subjective realism), 154; and breath of life, 44; and Christian contemplative tradition, 46, 170–72; and evil and free will in Judeo-Christian tradition, 53–56; and Hindu philosophy, 194; and human nature, 169; and Kabbalah, 193; Kant on, 155; and karma, 107; and metaphysical realism, 153, 189; Nicholas of Cusa on, 173, 180, 193–94; Origen on, 102; and personal identity in the Bible, 3–4

goodness, 3–4, 34–35, 53–56, 174, 176, 177

Great Perfection (Dzogchen) school of Tibetan Buddhism: and enlightenment, 179, 181–83; and life force, 179–80; meditation practice, 57–58, 181–82; and the nature of reality, 179–86, 194–95; parables on ultimate reality, 182–83; and Primordial Buddha, 194–95; and primordial consciousness, 179–85, 194–95; and substrate consciousness, 93, 195

Greek contemplative tradition: and death, 99–100; Neoplatonism, 10–11, 172, 193; orientation of meditation practice, 13; possible influence on Judeo-Christian tradition, 9–10; Pythagoras and, 7–9 (*see also* Pythagoras and Pythagoreans); and reincarnation, 8–11; *theoria,* 7, 11, 63

Greek Orthodox contemplative tradition, 44–45, 56, 58–59, 75–76

Greek philosophy: Epicurus, 54–55; Neoplatonism, 10, 172, 193; Plato, 10–83, 116; Plotinus, 10–11; Socrates, 10, 96, 99–100. *See also* Pythagoras and Pythagoreans

Greene, Karl, 111

Gregory of Nyssa, Saint, 170

Gregory Palamas, Saint, 45, 76, 170–71

ground of becoming, 89–90, 174–76
Guth, Alan, 191

happiness: Augustine on, 58, 83; Buddha on, 125, 145; Charvaka on, 54; and early Christianity, 46; emotional health, 4, 32–35, 42–44, 60–61; Freud on, 54; and gamma waves in the brain, 31; and lifestyle supportive of meditative practice, 64; and mind training (*lojong*), 145; Plotinus on, 10–11; similarities and differences in Buddhist and Christian views on, 59. *See also* bliss
Harvard Medical School, 27–28, 29
Hasidic tradition of Judaism, 104
Hawking, Stephen, 164–65, 191
health benefits of meditation, 29–36, 42–44, 60–61
heaven, 103, 169–74, 176
hell, 103
heresies, Christian, 103
Hertog, Thomas, 164–65
Hesychios the Priest, 75
Hindu philosophy, 54, 79, 101, 194. *See also* India
hospice care, 29–30
hostility, 64, 84, 140, 142, 146, 177
humanity, future of, 195–96

identity: Buddhist conception of necessary conditions for emergence of human psyche, 104, 117–18; and Buddhist self-less universe concept, 139–46; and evolution of the universe, 195; God and personal identity in Hindu philosophy, 194; and Great Perfection teachings, 195; happiness and liberation and the boundaries of the self, 59; and inversion of consciousness meditation, 82; mental events distinguished from self, 68; Merrell-Wolff's experiences in transcending personal identity, 79–80, 192; and the nature of reality, 145–46, 152; and primordial consciousness, 182–83; quest

for, 3; and suffering, 142–46; and Taylor on objects of scientific study, 156. *See also* soul
illusion. *See* delusion; reality, nature of
India: Charvaka's philosophy, 54; and the nature of reality, 139–40; and origins of Greek contemplative tradition, 8–9; pre-Buddhist tradition of contemplation, 11–12, 43, 80, 83–86; and reincarnation, 12–13, 100; and *samadhi*, 83–86; Shankara's formulation of Hindu philosophy, 79; three approaches to knowledge, 154. *See also* Buddhism; Buddhist contemplative tradition; Hindu philosophy; Mahayana Buddhism; Theravada Buddhism
inflationary universe, 191
information and meaning, 158–65; reincarnation, 108
insomnia, 29
introspection, 61–65; and artificial intelligence, 134; confusion over term, 91; defined/described, 63–64; James on, 20, 24, 68, 113; and mindfulness of awareness, 73
Islam, 11

James, William, 27; and beginnings of Western psychology, 20–21; and consciousness, 77; and introspection, 20, 24, 68, 113; models of brain–mind relationship, 96; and radical empiricism, 155; and scientific ignorance about consciousness, 125
Jesus: and breath of life, 44; as enlightened being, 177; Jesus prayer, 44, 48, 49; on love of God, 46; and possible Greek influences on early Christianity, 9–10; and rebirth, 102; resurrection of, 185–86; and salvation, 169–70
Jha, Amishi, 32
jiva, 94, 100, 108, 180–81. *See also* life force
Jiva Project (proposed), 117
jñana, 167, 179–85
John the Baptist, 9–10, 102
John of the Cross, Saint, 45, 170

Josephus, Flavius, 9–10, 101–2

Judaism: and breath of life, 44; Essenes, 9–10; evil and suffering in Judeo-Christian tradition, 53–56; Hasidic tradition, 104; Kabbalah, 104, 193; and the nature of reality, 193; and Origen, 11; Pharisees, 101–2; and Putnam, 156–57; and Pythagoras, 9; and reincarnation, 10, 101–2, 104; Sadducees, 102. See also Bible

Jung, Carl, 112

Justinian, Emperor, 103

Kabat-Zinn, Jon, 30–31

Kabbalah, 104, 193

Kant, Immanuel, 79, 155

karma, 104, 105, 107, 108

Keating, Thomas, 56

Kemeny, Margaret, 33

Kepler, 172

Khenpo Achö, 185–86

Koch, Christof, 66, 127

Laird, Martin, 56, 76–77, 170

Lamme, Victor A. F., 127–28

laxity, as attentional imbalance, 63–64, 73, 84, 177

Leon, Moses De, 104

life: meaning of, 46, 54; origin of, 121–22, 128–31

life force, 94; concept in 19th-century Western science, 121–22; and death, 184; in Great Perfection teachings, 179–80; memories stored in, 94, 115, 117; and reincarnation, 100, 108, 117

Linde, Andre, 190–91

loving-kindness, 174, 176

Lozang Chökyi Gyaltsen, 57, 81, 93

lucid dreaming, 88, 116

lucid dreamless sleep, 116

lucid dying, 94, 108

luminosity: and bhavanga (ground of becoming), 89; and the nature of reality, 149; and primordial consciousness, 167–68; as

quality of consciousness, 89; and substrate consciousness, 91–92

Luria, Isaac, 104

Macarius the Elder, 44

Machik Labkyi Drönma, 81

Mahakassapa, 100

Mahayana Buddhism: and bodhisattva way of life, 46, 176–77, 192; buddha nature, 176–78; Diamond Cutter Sutra, 146–47; and illusion, 146–47; and inversion of consciousness, 80–82; and life force, 94; and nirvana, 181; and samadhi, 85; settling the mind in its natural state exercise, 57

Maitripa, 57, 81

malice. See hostility

Mañjushrimitra, 178

mantras, 43, 44, 48, 49

Mary Magdalene, 185

Massachusetts General Hospital, 31

mathematics, 8–9, 18–19

Matt, Daniel C., 193

matter. See reality, nature of

Maximus the Confessor, 44

MBSR. See Mindfulness-Based Stress Reduction (MBSR) program

McGill University, 28–29

medication, and suffering, 55

meditation: attentional imbalances and hindrances, 63–64, 84–85, 177; awareness of consciousness meditation, 71–73, 79–88; and daily life, 64–65, 187–88; defined/described, 7–8; emptiness of matter meditation, 151–52; emptiness of mind meditation, 137–38; and enlightenment, 177; Great Perfection sequence, 181–82; health benefits of, 29–36, 42–44, 60–61; lack of scientific interest in contemplative inquiry, 16, 21–22, 25, 113, 132; mantras, 43, 44, 48, 49; and memory of past lives, 108–9; mindfulness meditation (see mindfulness meditation); and the nature of the observer, 87–88;

meditation (*continued*)

"nonmeditation" practice, 167–68; observing the mind, 48–51, 56–61, 65–69; oscillating awareness meditation, 97; Perfection of Wisdom meditation, 148–49; relation between meditation and contemplation, 7–8; resting in the stillness of awareness, 119; *samadhi* (see *samadhi*); scientific studies of, 27–36; and sense of personal identity, 141–42; settling the mind in its natural state exercise, 47–51, 61–63, 65–69; *shamatha* (meditative quiescence), 85, 92, 114; word origin, 15. *See also* Buddhist contemplative tradition; Christian contemplative tradition; Greek contemplative tradition; mindfulness meditation

memory: of interval between death and rebirth, 109–10; and last moments of life, 100–101; location of, 94, 115, 117; and mindfulness, 62–64; of past lives, 103, 105, 107–9, 114, 116

Menander I, 62

mental events: lack of means of examining in Western cognitive science, 24–25, 67, 78; location of, 66; neural correlates of, 24, 65, 127–28; nonphysical nature of, 22, 67–68, 131, 158; observing the mind, 48–51, 56–61, 65–69; and substrate, 94, 95–96; transition from egocentric to naturalistic view of mental phenomena, 61

Merrell-Wolff, Franklin, 79–81, 192

metaphysical realism, 153, 155–56, 189–90

Miller, Stanley, 121, 130

mind: and causes of suffering, 55–56; as emergent property, 23–24, 54, 122–23; location of, 65–69; observing the mind, 48–51, 56–69; and role of the observer in experimental physics, 160–62, 191–92; self-healing capacity of, 44, 60–61; settling the mind in its natural state, 47–51, 60–61, 65–69; sign of the mind, 89–90. *See also* consciousness; identity; mental events; mind–brain

relationship; subconscious mind; substrate consciousness

Mind and Life Institute, 35

mind–brain relationship: and causality, 23–24, 55; James's models of, 96; and location of the mind, 65–66; and neuroscience, 5, 22–23, 65–66, 122–23; and reincarnation, 105–6; and sense of personal identity, 142; and substrate, 95–96; and Wheeler's hypothesis on information, 162–63

mindfulness meditation, 42–44, 61–65; and Buddhism, 43–44, 62–65; and Christian contemplative tradition, 44–45; and memory of past lives, 105; mindfulness defined/described, 61, 63–64; mindfulness of awareness, 71–73; mindfulness of breathing exercise, 39–40, 42–44; and stress reduction, 30–32, 42–44

Mindfulness-Based Stress Reduction (MBSR) program, 30–31

Moggallana, 84

monasticism, 11

Nagasena, 62–63

natural disasters, 108

near-death experiences, 110–11

Neoplatonism, 10, 172, 193

neuroscience: assumptions of, 23, 78, 96, 122–23; assumptions about future accomplishments of, 130, 158–59; conclusions about consciousness predetermined by limitations of methods of inquiry, 132; emotions and suffering, 55; epigenetics, 28–29; inability to detect consciousness, 78, 123–25, 127, 131; incompleteness of, 5, 23, 65–66, 122–23, 125; neural correlates of mental processes, 24, 65, 127–28; neurogenesis, 28–29; neuroplasticity studies, 27–28. *See also* mental events; mind–brain relationship; skepticism

Newton, Isaac, 189

Nicholas of Cusa, 172–74, 180, 192–94

quantum cosmology, 190–91
quantum field theory, 159
quantum mechanics, 66, 129; and closure principle, 159; and consciousness, 189–91; and Hawking and Hertog's ideas on cosmology, 164–65; and role of the observer, 160–62, 190–91

rainbow body, 183–85
reality, nature of: Berkeley on, 154; and buddha nature, 177; Buddhist discourse on illusion, 146–50, 152; and Buddhist emphasis on direct perception, 154–55; Buddhist self-less universe concept, 139–46; chariot metaphor, 144–46; Charvaka on, 54; co-creation of reality, 156–58, 162, 191, 197–98; and conservation of consciousness, 95–96; contemplative inquiry as tool for exploring, 7–8, 15; cosmology, 164–65, 190–95; and dependent origination, 144–45, 150; Descartes on, 18–19, 65–67; and empiricism, 153–57; Epicurus on, 54; and Great Perfection teachings, 179–86; information and meaning, 158–65; and Jewish mysticism, 193; and karma, 108; and metaphysical realism, 153, 155–56, 189; and modern physics, 66, 129, 158–65, 189–91; Nicholas of Cusa on, 193–94; and perfect symmetry, 189–92; and personal identity, 145–46, 152; Plotinus on, 10; pre-Buddhist Indian concepts, 139–40; Putnam on, 156–57; and substrate, 94, 149–50, 152
refractory period following emotionally disturbing experience, 34–35
reincarnation, 99–118; and biological evidence, 116–17; Buddhist contemplative inquiry into, 113–15; Buddhist views on, 104–5, 108–9; and contemplative scientific research into consciousness, 113–18; craving as impetus for, 101; cycle of amnesia, 116; Evagrius of Pontus and, 11; and India, 12–13; interval between death and rebirth, 101, 109–10; in Judeo-Christian tradition, 10–11,

101–4; of lamas in Tibetan Buddhism, 109, 117; and life force (*jiva*), 100; memory of past lives, 103, 105, 107–9, 114, 116; and near-death experiences, 110–11; Plotinus and, 10–11; Pythagoras and, 8–9, 99–100, 101; scientific resistance to concept, 99, 106, 112; scientific studies of, 105–13; Socrates and, 99–100; and substrate, 94
religion, 15; faith-based religion and the rise of modern science, 15–18, 189; faith-based religion distinguished from experiential spirituality, 2, 12, 15, 105, 125; and taboo against subjective experience in science, 22; and traditional hierarchy of scientific inquiry, 112
The Republic (Plato), 116
Reynolds, Pam, 110–11
robotics, 123–24, 126
Roman Catholic contemplative tradition, 58–59
Russian Orthodox contemplative tradition, 76

Sadducees, 102
Salk Institute for Biological Studies, 28
samadhi, 82–86; and Buddha's studies, 12; and death, 100; defined/described, 84; degrees of, 84–86; and inversion of consciousness, 80; and memory of past lives, 105; and nirvana, 85; and reincarnation, 113–14; and *shamatha,* 85; and substrate, 94–95
Samantabhadra, 194–95
Santa Barbara Institute for Consciousness Studies, 35–36, 114–15
Sartre, Jean-Paul, 42
sati, 62–65. See also mindfulness meditation
Saxena, Hanumant, 107
Schrödinger wave equation, 190–91
science: and Christianity, 15–18, 189; conclusions about consciousness predetermined by limitations of methods of inquiry, 132; contemplative skepticism about scientific approaches to biology and consciousness, 128–35; and Descartes, 18–19; Feynman on

progress in, 135; and Galileo, 17–19; lack of authentic science of consciousness, 77–78; marginalization of inward-looking contemplative inquiry, 16, 21–22, 25, 113, 132; materialism (*see* scientific materialism); and Nicholas of Cusa's threefold approach to knowledge, 172–74; origins of modern science, 15–19, 189; origins of Western psychology, 20–21; parallels between evolution of human knowledge and beliefs about evolution of the cosmos, 163–64; Putnam on philosophy of science, 157; and reincarnation, 99, 105–13; science's inability to detect consciousness, 78, 123–25, 127, 131, 133, 164; scientific method, 17–18, 24; scientism, 129; Taylor on objects of scientific study, 156; traditional hierarchy of scientific inquiry, 112; word origin, 19. *See also* biology; cognitive science; contemplative inquiry, scientific; neuroscience; physics; skepticism

scientific materialism: assumptions about death, 99; assumptions about future accomplishments, 130, 158–59; definition of the physical, 159; James and, 113; and origins of life, 121–22, 130, 131; rejection of inexplicable phenomena, 183; and skepticism, 121–25; and traditional hierarchy of scientific inquiry, 112–13

Searle, John R., 126–27

self. *See* identity; soul

sensory perception: and breath of life exercise, 40; and craving and hostility, 64; Descartes on, 18–19, 66–67; and empiricism, 150; and the nature of reality, 154–58; Nicholas of Cusa on, 172–74; and substrate consciousness, 92

sentient beings, 92, 161; and buddha nature, 196; welfare of all sentient beings, 46, 176, 177, 181, 192

shamatha, 85, 92, 114

Shamatha Project, 114–15

Shankara, 79

Shantideva, 177

Shimon Bar Yochai, 104

skepticism, 121–35; contemplative skepticism, 125, 128–35 (*see also* religion: faith-based religion distinguished from experiential spirituality); philosophical skepticism, 125–28; scientific skepticism, 121–25

Skinner, B. F., 125–27

sleep: and ground of becoming, 90, 174; and substrate, 94, 150, 152; and substrate consciousness, 93

social sciences, and unwritten hierarchy of scientific inquiry, 112

Socrates, 10, 96, 99–100

soul: Anan teen David on, 104; Augustine on, 58, 83, 103; and Christian contemplative tradition, 58–59; and death, 99 (*see also* reincarnation); Epicurus on, 54; and faith-based religion, 15; in modern Christianity, 102–5, 190; Origen on, 102; and substrate consciousness, 93. *See also* identity

Sources of the Self (Taylor), 156

space: absolute space of phenomena, 177, 179–81, 184, 194; excitations of, 159; and substrate, 94, 149, 162; and symmetry-breaking in the early universe, 191

Spetzler, Robert, 110–11

Steindl-Rast, David, 185

Stevenson, Ian, 107–8, 112, 117

stress reduction, 29–34, 43–44

subconscious mind, 4, 49, 51, 69, 91

subjective idealism, 154

subjectivity: insights gained from meditation, 5 (*see also* consciousness; reality, nature of; suffering); left out of Western psychology and neuroscience, 5, 16, 21–22, 25, 122–23, 125–27; and settling the mind in its natural state, 65–69

substrate, 94–95, 180–81; and memory, 94, 115; and modern physics, 159–60, 162; and the nature of reality, 149–50, 152; and Primordial Buddha, 195; and sleep, 150, 152